OCCUPATIONAL THERAPY FOR
STROKE REHABILITATION

THERAPY IN PRACTICE SERIES

Edited by Jo Campling

This series of books is aimed at 'therapists' concerned with rehabilation in a very broad sense. The intended audience particularly includes occupational therapists, physiotherapists and speech therapists, but many titles will also be of interest to nurses, psychologists, medical staff, social workers, teachers or voluntary workers. Some volumes are interdisciplinary, others are aimed at one particular profession. All titles will be comprehensive but concise, and practical but with due reference to relevant theory and evidence. They are not research monographs but focus on professional practice, and will be of value to both students and qualified personnel.

Occupational Therapy for Stroke Rehabilitation

SIMON B.N. THOMPSON and MARYANNE MORGAN

CHAPMAN & HALL

London · Glasgow · Weinheim · New York · Tokyo · Melbourne · Madras

Published by Chapman & Hall, 2-6 Boundary Row, London SE1 8HN, UK

Chapman & Hall, 2-6 Boundary Row, London SE1 8HN, UK

Blackie Academic & Professional, Wester Cleddens Road, Bishopbriggs, Glasgow G64 2NZ, UK

Chapman & Hall GmbH, Pappelallee 3, 69469 Weinheim, Germany

Chapman & Hall USA, One Penn Plaza, 41st Floor, New York, NY10119, USA

Chapman & Hall Japan, ITP - Japan, Kyowa Building, 3F, 2-2-1 Hirakawacho, Chiyoda-ku, Tokyo 102, Japan

Chapman & Hall Australia, Thomas Nelson Australia, 102 Dodds Street, South Melbourne, Victoria 3205, Australia

Chapman & Hall India, R. Seshadri, 32 Second Main Road, CIT East, Madras 600 035, India

First edition 1990
Reprinted 1995

© 1990 Simon B.N. Thompson and Maryanne Morgan

Typeset in 10/12pt Times by Leaper & Gard Ltd, Bristol
Printed in Great Britain by St Edmundsbury Press, Suffolk

ISBN 0 412 33530 1

A Catalogue record for this book is available from the British Library
Library of Congress Cataloging-in-Publication Data
Thompson, Simon.   Occupational therpay for stroke rehabilitation/
Simon Thompson and Maryanne Morgan.
        p.   cm. - (Therapy in practice series:11)
    Includes bibliographical references.
    ISBN 0-412-33530-1
    1. Cerebrovascular disease-Patients-Rehabilitation.
2. Occupational therapy.   I. Morgan, Maryanne, 1959-
II. Title. III. Series.
    [DNLM: 1. Cerebrovascular Disorders-rehabilitation.
2. Occupational Therapy.   WL355 T476o]
RC388.5.T475   1990
616.8'1-dc20
DNLM/DLC
for Library of Congress   89-23989
                                                          CIP

Contents

Acknowledgements

The authors would like to thank the following: Kevin Cook for all his hard work; Mike Coleman and Annie Turner for their encouragement and advice; Avril Drummond, Judy Edmans and Carole Roberts for advice on the occupational therapy application; Sue Croshaw for typing; Fiona Sidgwick for proof reading; and of course, to our parents for their continuing support.

Preface

This book is both an introductory text to the rehabilitation of stroke for student therapists and a reference text for qualified therapists. The layout of the book reflects these needs with Chapters 1–4 assuming a minimal level of understanding of the material. These chapters provide an introduction to the condition of stroke itself, the problem therapists face in assessing and treating stroke patients and therapeutic approaches in occupational therapy. Prognosis of stroke is also discussed which is an issue taken up in later chapters concerned with expert systems.

The use of microcomputers in occupational therapy is discussed throughout the book with particular reference to their direct role during therapy. Chapters 5–7 assume a higher level of understanding from the reader although students will find the material useful as an insight into the work of the modern-day therapist. Chapter 5 addresses the work carried out in the area of biofeedback; Chapter 6 introduces the concept and uses of databases, and Chapter 7 discusses the versatility of microcomputers, especially in the provision of expert systems for the prognosis of stroke.

A comprehensive Glossary, Reference section and Index provide information for all levels of use which complements other books in the Therapy in Practice series. It is hoped that this book will be informative for those who require more than just a basic knowledge of stroke rehabilitation. As information technology is becoming increasingly important in all areas of therapy, this information is essential to ensure the continuing growth of the profession.

Introduction

Occupational therapy involves the diagnosis, assessment, treatment and prognosis of patients suffering from conditions such as stroke. In the 1980s therapists concerned with the rehabilitation of stroke victims recognized the benefits of information technology, in particular microcomputers, applied to each of these areas. The importance of this recognition has been reflected by the use and development of both hardware and software (e.g. 'concept keyboards' and programs to improve motor and cognitive function).

Therapists were initially encouraged to introduce information technology into their departments under the DHSS/DTI Scheme in 1983. This involved the issue of BBC B Microcomputers to several rehabilitation units for research and experimentation.

The benefits of using information technology in rehabilitation departments are numerous. For example, microcomputers not only save time and space storing medical data in databases, but they can also provide accurate and fast records of direct physiological measurements. Similarly, long and complicated data manipulations (e.g. retrieving data according to a particular category or making a mathematical calculation) can be made very quickly and often far more efficiently than by therapists.

However, inherent with these benefits are some disadvantages. Microcomputers can be relatively costly and are prone to human error. To avoid information being lost, backup procedures such as printouts and disc copies are required. There is also the need for therapists to be familiar with the new technology. It is not necessary for therapists to be computer programmers, but there is a need to have a basic knowledge of computing to meet the requirements of their patients and environment.

Most therapists and clinicians using information technology agree that the problems of using microcomputers are far outweighed by the advantages; they offer a new and exciting contribution to many areas of patient care, especially to the rehabilitation of stroke.

1

Epidemiology

DEFINITIONS OF STROKE

Stroke, also referred to as cerebrovascular accident (CVA) has been defined by the World Health Organization (WHO) as:

> . . . rapidly developing clinical signs of cerebral function, lasting more than 24 hours or leading to death, with no apparent cause other than of vascular origin' (Aho *et al.*, 1980).

Indeed, this definition is widely used as a reference in writings on this subject. However, the National Survey of Stroke in the United States of America used a longer but more specific definition:

> Stroke is a clinical syndrome consisting of a constellation of neurological findings, sudden or rapid in onset, which persist for more than 24 hours and whose vascular origins are limited to:
>
> (a) Thrombotic or embolic occlusion of a cerebral artery resulting in infarction, or;
> (b) Spontaneous rupture of a vessel resulting in intracerebral or subarachnoid haemorrhage.'

It should be noted that this definition excludes occlusion or rupture due to traumatic, neoplastic, or infectious processes which produce vascular pathology.

Another definition commonly referred to is:

A cerebrovascular accident (CVA or stroke) is a sudden attack of weakness affecting one side of the body, resulting from an interruption to the flow of blood to the brain (by thrombosis, embolus, or ruptured aneurysm). A stroke can vary in severity from a weakness in a limb with some perceptual problems to a profound paralysis and considerable impairment (Isaacs, 1983; Thompson, 1987a).

It is important to realize the consequences of these definitions and to understand the two central features linking them; i.e. the sudden rapid onset (which has a devastating effect on the stroke victim) and the site of disturbance — the brain (the central control system for the whole body).

Epidemiological studies tend to use the WHO definition but some clinical studies may be less strict. This can lead to problems when considering a variety of studies for discussion.

AETIOLOGY

A stroke is caused by anoxia (lack of oxygen) to the vital tissues of the central nervous system; i.e. the brain cells. The blood supply to the brain (Figures 1.1 and 1.2) can be affected most commonly by the following:

1. Cerebral haemorrhage. This occurs when a weakness in the artery wall, or trauma to the vessel causes sudden bleeding into the brain tissue. The build-up of pressure caused by the increased volume of blood around the cells causes damage by bruising or by a reduction in the supply of oxygen to the cells;
2. Cerebral infarction. This is when permanent death of cells occurs due to cerebral haemorrhage. Permanent functional deficit associated with the affected area of the cortex may ensue;

3. Cerebral embolism or thrombus. A thrombus is a collection (or clot) of blood cells or other matter in the lining of the artery. This eventually blocks the arterial supply to the tissues that the artery supplies. If this occurs in the blood vessels supplying the brain, the oxygen and nutritional supply will be cut off and a stroke may follow. Alternatively, a small piece of the thrombus may break away and form an embolus (a travelling clot of blood) which will lodge in the smaller vessels, thereby having the same effect of preventing oxygen from penetrating the brain cells.

Figure 1.1 The origin of the intracranial arteries from the aorta. Olf., olfactory tract; MS, medial striate artery; LS, lateral striate artery; ACh., anterior choroidal artery; MC, middle cerebral artery; 3, cranial nerve 3; mb, midbrain; u, uncus; IC, internal carotid artery; V, vertebral artery; MED, medulla; EC, external carotid artery; CC, common carotid artery; S, subclavian artery; A, aorta. (From *Clinical Neuroanatomy made Ridiculously Simple*, Goldberg, 1983.)

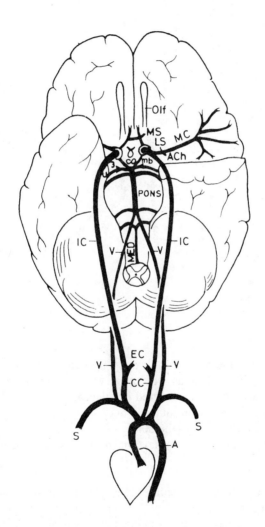

Figure 1.2 The major arterial supply to the brain.
ACA, anterior cerebral artery; MCA, middle cerebral artery; PCA,
posterior cerebral artery; PAD, pia, arachnoid, dura. (From *Clinical
Neuroanatomy made Ridiculously Simple*, Goldberg, 1983.)

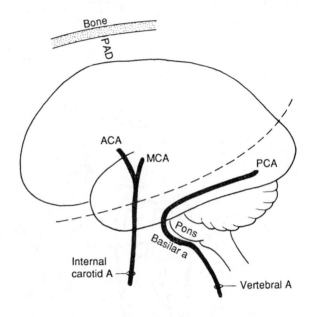

The brain is the most complex organ of the body, and as such,
damage to different areas will cause varying functional deficits.
Brain cells are usually considered irreplaceable compared to other
tissue areas that can reproduce as necessary. However, the possibilities of brain plasticity (the ability of brain cells to take over the
function of damaged areas) have been investigated (Bach-y-Rita,
1981):

1. Sprouting. Numerous studies have confirmed that brain cells
    have the capacity to sprout and this may have an important
    impact on recovery following damage (Raisman and Field,
    1973). With sprouting, new cells are formed which take over
    the function of the damaged cells;

2. Unmasking. Nerve cells can adjust their excitability to maintain full function when some of the inputs are lost (Wall, 1980). Wall (1980) considered that there are suppressed connections that come into play when damage occurs.

This ability of brain cells to sprout or unmask can be seen where stroke patients may have extreme difficulty in performing a specific movement early on, but this movement becomes possible at a later time (Bach-y-Rita, 1980).

ACUTE STROKE

The effects of stroke

Physical effects

A stroke can affect a person in many ways. For example, dysphagia (difficulty with swallowing) is extremely distressing to the patient and relatives who may be assisting with early encouragement in feeding (Selley, 1985). If the patient's nutritional and liquid needs are not met, there can be a deterioration in the general health of the patient resulting in slower or impaired recovery.

Incontinence, whether through specific neurological problems or lack of mobility, is humiliating. It all contributes to the indignity felt by many patients in hospital. Reassurance and routine-setting are essential features of the early management of stroke.

Sensory (or motor) loss resulting in hemiplegia (paralysis of one half of the body) or hemiparesis (partial paralysis of one half of the body) with or without hemianasthesia (sensory loss of the half that is paralysed), is the most common motor problem following stroke. One side of the body, including the face, may be completely or partially paralysed leading to poor mobility, loss of balance and control of limbs, slumping posture and lack of sensation. Sensory loss may lead to trapping or dragging of limbs as well as skin damage due to lack of awareness of painful stimuli.

Communication

In all areas of communication close work with the speech therapist will be advantageous. Speech therapists will carry out their own

5

assessment, and will work with other disciplines to maintain a consistent approach to the patient.

Dysphasia is a language deficit caused by damage to the speech centre of the brain and can be expressive or receptive. Expressive dysphasia means the patient will have difficulty conversing in a sensible format; words may be mispronounced, or whole sentences may be non-sensical. In these cases it is essential to remember that despite the expressive problems the patient is likely to be able to comprehend perfectly adequately what is being said. This is the opposite case in receptive dysphasia. In this instance the patient may not understand the spoken or written word and a communication system using symbols or gestures needs to be established.

Dysarthria may be another problem encountered with communication impairment. This is where speech articulation is reduced usually by the paralysis of one side of the mouth and tongue. In these cases careful listening skills are required to verify the patient's requests.

Cognition

Confusion following a stroke, especially in the elderly, can be difficult to resolve. Patients who are unaware of time or space orientation may become distressed if they cannot understand where they are, or their purpose in that particular place. This may lead to wandering, difficulty in finding the way home, or a lack of recognition of visitors or staff.

Memory loss is frustrating and can be dangerous in the home setting if not recognized and taken into account (e.g. leaving cookers on or unattended). Memory loss also slows down the rehabilitation process as patients cannot remember the sequence of tasks. Similarly, re-learning can be much more difficult.

Behavioural problems such as swearing, shouting, attempts to abscond (possibly resulting in falls) can be frustrating for carers, whether in hospital or at home. These problems may stem from confusion and a lack of understanding of the situation or as a result of language deficits where the patient is unaware of the abusive nature of his/her attempts at communication.

Concentration if poor (as it often will be in the early days when fatigue and general malaise may be affecting the patient) can impede rehabilitation from stroke. There is a need to break down tasks into small stages of achievement as well as grade them in time. For example a patient cannot be expected to completely dress him/herself at once but some assistance may be given at each stage to enable completion of the task as a whole.

Perception

Early problems identified in this area will be neglect of the affected side shown by posture and the patient's inability to recognize his/her own limbs. The upper limb is usually the most problematical as it may be left hanging over the chair leading to subluxation of the shoulder (where the head of the humerus drops out of the glenoid cavity due to laxity of ligaments and lack of tone on the surrounding muscles).

Hemianopia is a visual perceptual deficit that may be noticed especially when the patient is beginning to feed or dress him/herself. The patient may leave half a plate of food or only attempt to wash or dress the unaffected half of the body. This would be highlighted later in more specific perceptual testing.

Emotion

Emotional lability, fear and denial of disability are examples of common psychological problems in the early stages of stroke often coupled with confusion. Inappropriate laughter or crying can be very disconcerting to other ward patients and relatives. This needs to be treated with patience and tolerance as the patient will usually be unaware of his/her plight. Fear of the future, which often leads to denial of any problem, can also occur and again requires reassurance, explanation and a sympathetic approach.

More severe psychological effects such as anxiety, agitation, or clinical depression, require more specific intervention. A patient who is severely depressed will lack motivation to perform even the simplest tasks (such as maintaining posture, attempting communication, etc.). (Ebrahim, 1985; Collin, Tinson and Lincoln, 1987). Similarly, a patient who is over-anxious or extremely agitated will not be able to settle to the routine and demands of the rehabilitation programme. In these cases psychiatric assessment and treatment (leading to the possible use of drugs) enables the continuation of the rehabilitation process.

FAMILY INVOLVEMENT

The initial shock felt by the whole family of the stroke victim is very real and alarming. The family may feel helpless, convinced that their loved one is going to die and may not appreciate all that is going on around them (Fisher, 1961; Borden, 1962).

The therapist and staff involved in the rehabilitation process can assist in the very early stages by giving clear explanations of procedures, positioning and treatment techniques.

Rapport-building between the patient and relatives can commence on the ward and will greatly assist co-operation during the prolonged period of hospitalization and rehabilitation. It is also very important to involve the spouse in the treatment regime so that they can continue activities in a consistent manner, for example, by showing pictures or 'get-well' cards to the affected side, assisting with feeding, drinking, washing and dressing activities, etc. This will enable the spouse to see what abilities the patient has and to see the progress for themselves. This can be extremely comforting and rewarding for both the patient and the spouse.

At a later stage support groups for relatives may be introduced depending on either the spouse or the patient's individual needs or expressed desires. This will enable them to receive more information and make contact with others in similar situations. It has been shown that both patients, relatives and staff find such meetings beneficial (Mykyta *et al.*, 1976).

INCIDENCE OF STROKE

This is the number of new cases that occur in a defined population in a given period. In western countries, 150–250 people in every 100 000 may be expected to have a stroke (Aho *et al.*, 1980). More specifically, in the UK, 200 in every 100 000 are likely to have a stroke (Oxfordshire Community Stroke Project, 1983) compared to 500 in 100 000 who suffer from myocardial infarction (a type of heart attack); more than double that of stroke. Indeed, stroke is the third most frequent cause of death next to ischaemic heart disease and cancer.

However, the true incidence of stroke is very hard to establish as 38–60% of patients with stroke never attend hospital. To overcome this it has been suggested that a community register of stroke occurrence would be more realistic as an indicator of incidence (Barnford *et al.*, 1986).

Between the sexes, men suffer with stroke more than women, a difference more pronounced in middle age but reducing in old age. It is thought that the protective effect of hormones in women in preventing arterial disease may afford some explanation of this as the incidence of stroke in women increases after the menopause to almost match that of men.

As might be expected the incidence of stroke increases with age as shown in table 1.1. This table shows the incidence of stroke related to age as evidenced in the *Oxfordshire Stroke Project* (1983).

Recurrence

Every year approximately 10% of survivors from stroke will suffer a recurrent stroke. Figure 1.3 shows the degree to which death and disability will prevail in the first year following the stroke. The scales used are the modified Rankin Disability Scales shown in table 1.2 (Dennis and Warlow, 1987).

RISK FACTORS

Definition of risk factors

What is meant by risk factors? Risk factors are certain characteristics that give an increased likelihood of a stroke occurring. They

Table 1.1
Incidence of stroke related to age
(Oxfordshire Stroke Project, 1983)

Age group	Incidence (per 1000 pop. per year)
35–44	0.25
45–54	1.00
55–64	3.50
65–74	9.00
75–84	20.00
85+	40.00

Figure 1.3 Percentage of stroke victims who are independent (Rankin scale 0-2); dependent (Rankin scale 3-5); and dead, one year following stroke. (From Dennis and Warlow, 1987.)

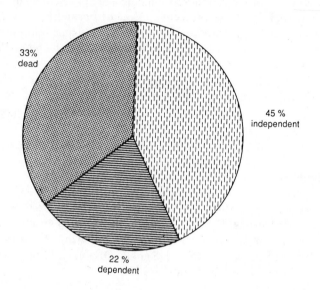

33%
dead

45 %
independent

22 %
dependent

Table 1.2
Modified Rankin disability scale
(from Dennis and Warlow, 1987)

0	No symptoms
1	Minor symptoms that do not interfere with lifestyle
2	Minor disability symptoms that lead to some restriction of lifestyle, but do not interfere with patients' capacity to look after themselves
3	Moderate disability symptoms that significantly restrict the lifestyle and/or prevent totally independent existence
4	Moderately severe disability: symptoms that prevent independent existence though not needing constant attention
5	Severe disability, totally dependent, requiring constant attention day and night

fall into three areas: relative risk, absolute risk, and attributable risk (Wade *et al.*, 1985). Relative risk is the increase in risk associated with possession of a certain characteristic compared with a similar person lacking that characteristic; absolute risk is the rate at which people possessing a characteristic will actually have a stroke; and attributable risk indicates the proportion of strokes caused by the characteristic. Some examples to illustrate these types of risk factors are:

1. The contraceptive pill. A person taking the contraceptive pill has an increased relative risk of stroke three times higher than that of someone who is not taking it but since the group of people actually taking the pill is so small and specific (i.e. younger women) the absolute risk in the population is extremely small;
2. Bacterial endocarditis. Patients with this condition have a high relative risk and absolute risk of having a stroke but as the condition is so rare the attributable risk to the population is negligible.

Risk factor significance

The following is an attempt to place risk factors in some order of significance for the incidence of strokes:

1. Hypertension;
2. Cardiac disease
   atrial fibrillation
   Ischaemic heart disease (IHD);
3. Cerebrovascular disease: Transient ischaemic attacks (TIA);
4. Diabetes mellitus;
5. Hyperlipidaemia;
6. Smoking;
7. Contraceptive pill;
8. Other causes
   stress
   diet
   alcohol
   climate
   physical activity
   seasonal variations in temperature.

Hypertension

The association between hypertension (high blood pressure) and stroke is well known (Cressman and Gifford, 1983). It is said to be the single most important risk factor possibly accounting for 70% of strokes with the risk increasing considerably with higher blood pressure. However, there is some question as to whether the treatment of hypertension reduces the risk of stroke or whether in some cases especially the elderly with mild hypertension, there is a danger of increasing the risk (Kannel and Wolf, 1983; Jansen *et al.*, 1986).

Cardiac disease

The Framingham study discovered that over 75% of stroke victims also had some form of cardiac disease (Kannel and Wolf, 1983). Indeed, it should be remembered that although stroke and cardiac disease are two separate illnesses they are linked by arteriosclerosis (the narrowing of the arteries) which is common to both. Examples of cardiac disease are:

1. Atrial fibrillation. This is present in 15% of stroke patients (Sandercock, 1984). This relative risk of stroke increases six times if associated with rheumatic disease (Kannel and Wolf, 1983);
2. Ischaemic heart disease (IHD). There is an increased risk of stroke with IHD due to the association with atheroma (thickening) of the arteries to the brain (Dennis and Warlow, 1987).

Cerebrovascular disease

It may seem obvious that cerebrovascular disease is considered a risk factor for stroke but perhaps less obvious are the risk factors concerned with transient ischaemic attacks (TIA). Of those people suffering from TIA up to 30% are at risk of suffering a stroke within two years, half of these within the first twelve months (Herman, Layten, van Luijk *et al.*, 1982a; Whisnant, 1974; Kannel and Wolf, 1983). TIA can easily be confused with cerebrovascular disease initially but as the term suggests, these attacks are transient and the patient recovers quickly. To reduce the risk of stroke the patient may take aspirin (reduces the risk by 20%) or have surgery such as carotid endarterectomy although the value of this is still unproven (Dennis and Warlow, 1987; Harrison and Dyken, 1983).

There have been various incidence studies regarding the rate of risk of cerebrovascular disease with results varying between 18% (Aho *et al.*, 1980), 26% (Walker *et al.*, 1981) and as high as 30% (Herman *et al.*, 1982a) although Kannel and Wolf (1983) suggest the average to be 10%.

Diabetes mellitus

Diabetes Mellitus is more common in stroke patients than in the normal population of a similar age. As there is a link between diabetes mellitus, hypertension and hyperlipidaemia it is difficult to assess which has the most effect on stroke. However, when all three conditions are present the relative risk of suffering a stroke is greater.

The Framingham study (Kannel and Wolf, 1983) showed that diabetics are more likely to suffer stroke (2.5 times for men and 3.7 times for women) and that for 10% of men and 14% of women the stroke was attributed to diabetes which also caused arterial disease.

Hyperlipidaemia

This is an excess of fat in the bloodstream which is known to be associated with the development of atheroma in coronary blood vessels. Therefore, this condition often occurs in patients suffering from hypertension. Again, it is difficult to assess whether stroke is due specifically to hyperlipidaemia or a combination of conditions that include hyperlipidaemia.

Smoking

The Framingham study (Kannel and Wolf, 1983) showed that the risk of stroke due to smoking was relatively small in people under 65 years of age and even less for people under 55 years. Most other studies (Herman *et al.*, 1982a) show little evidence of a link between smoking and an increased risk of stroke.

Contraceptive pill

As mentioned earlier the contraceptive pill is a relative risk factor but as the pill is only used by a small, specific part of the population the absolute risk is very small indeed (as low as 1 in 10000 people). The pill is thought to be a risk factor because of the effect it has in raising the blood pressure (Kannel and Wolf, 1983).

Other causes

It is often thought that stress is likely to precipitate a stroke but there is little evidence to prove this (Gentry *et al.*, 1979). Similarly diet, alcohol, climate, physical activity and temperature variations have all been studied but again there is little evidence of them having a significant effect on the incidence of stroke (Ashley, 1982; Hillbom and Kaste, 1983; Gill *et al.*, 1986).

PROGNOSIS AND OUTCOME

Variables affecting prognosis

The study of the prognosis of chronic disease is complicated by variations within and between patients in the course of a disease and by the fact that many factors may be associated with prognosis. The objective of therapeutic intervention is to increase the probability of favourable outcomes and to reduce the probability of unfavourable outcomes especially death (as many severe strokes result in death shortly afterwards). Such outcomes may be the occurrence of specific events such as death or occurrence of a stroke, or they may involve disease states which may be measured by continuous variables such as blood pressure or pulmonary function tests. It is important that the therapist has some awareness of the prognosis of the patient he/she treats. It is only by being aware of the probabilities of various complications and outcomes that adequate preventive measures and intervention with therapy may be taken.

When prognosis is expressed in such probabilistic terms it suggests that stochastic models (i.e. based on probabilities) may be a useful tool in the prognosis process (Smith, 1978). The first stochastic model used in the study of a chronic disease was that of Fix and Neyman (1951). Since their pioneering work several stochastic models have been used in the study of chronic diseases (Iosifescu and Tautu, 1973; Hill and Smith, 1974) but their full potential has not always been recognized (Smith, 1978). One application which has not been well documented is their use in the calculation of the prognosis of individual patients. Such an application is only practicable in the clinical setting if the prognosis can be obtained rapidly and without the need to refer to detailed tables. The developments of computer hardware are beginning to show clearer advances in this respect (Coe *et al.*, 1975), which has encouraged Thompson (1987f) to pursue this line of thought.

In considering the variables affecting prognosis the practising physician must often weigh the appropriateness for the patient of a dynamic short-term stay in a rehabilitation hospital as opposed to convalescence and gradual rehabilitation at a long-term care facility. This question is sometimes difficult to answer.

A retrospective study was made of the average improvement, length of stay and discharge placement of 180 stroke patients admitted to a rehabilitation hospital (Adler, Brown and Acton, 1980). Patients were divided into four age groups: under 55, 55–65, 66–75 and over 75. A grading system was used for evaluating the patient's ability in mobility and self-care. No significant differences were found among the four age groups. The patients were then divided into subgroups depending upon the admission function score: 0–20, 21–40, 41–60 and over 60.

In the subgroups no statistically significant differences were apparent for the average improvement of patients under 55 as compared to those over 75, except for those whose initial functional score was 21–40. In this subgroup the average improvement for patients under 55 was 26.4 points with a length of stay of 31.9 days, whereas for those over 75 the average improvement was 15.5 points with a length of stay of 25.9 days. Thus, age *per se* did not seem to be a determinant factor in successful rehabilitation; rather, the poor showing of the oldest group for the 21–40 score in the subset may have been due to premature discharge (Adler, Brown and Acton, 1980).

There are a number of variables that can influence the prognosis of a stroke patient and it is often difficult to isolate these individual variables in order to permit the most favourable outcome for the patient. In the end, with the aid of assessment charts, previous studies and statistics, it is the skill and experience of the combined treatment team that will determine the prognosis and subsequent course of treatment for an individual patient. Until the results of prognosis-related studies, such as computer-assisted feedback (Thompson, 1984a) can be confirmed by further research involving larger samples and a greater cross-section of patients, the prognosis team must continue to rely on their 'subjective' interpretation of the patient's condition.

Knowledge acquisition for a prognostic model of stroke

In order to discern which aspects of a patient's medical history may have contributed to his/her recovery it is necessary to firstly know the extent of disability and then to understand which anatomical sites affect function. Knowledge of such cerebral function and circulation greatly assists the occupational therapist in interpreting the symptomatology to determine the extent of the stroke and the area involved. For example, the functions normally associated with the frontal lobe are intellect, emotions, behaviour, language, personality, control centres for higher autonomic functions, abstract thinking, and motor movement (Goetter, 1986). The parietal lobe is responsible for reception, perception, and interpretation of sensory information including touch, pain, temperature, pressure, size, shape, and awareness of space (Rose and Capildeo, 1981; Sharpless, 1982). Alterations in blood flow through the internal carotid, middle cerebral, and anterior cerebral arteries produce dysfunction of the frontal and parietal lobes.

It is possible to differentiate between a stroke involving the anterior cerebral artery or one involving the middle cerebral artery by noting whether contralateral weakness, numbness, or paralysis is greater in the lower extremities than in the face and upper extremities. Lower extremity symptoms are associated with middle cerebral artery involvement while facial and upper extremity symptoms indicate anterior cerebral artery involvement. In addition, mental changes, dyspraxia, bowel and bladder incontinence, and alterations in grasping and sucking reflexes are associated with cerebral artery involvement. Symptomatology with internal carotid artery and middle cerebral artery involvement are similar and may include unilateral loss of vision, hemianopia, coma, aphasia, agnosia, and apraxia (Goetter, 1986). Therefore it is important to identify these factors in order to assess each patient's condition.

Precise interpretation of symptomatology is further dependent upon an understanding of the effect of cerebral dominance on function (Hart, 1983), which is particularly important to know for the rehabilitation of the stroke patient. Cerebral dominance refers

16

to the control that one hemisphere has over certain functions. It was believed that the cerebral dominance for language and handedness were related. However, research has shown that 80 or 90% of all individuals were found to have left hemisphere dominance for the understanding and expression of written language regardless of handedness (Rudy, 1984). Studies have shown cerebral dominance for other functions (Wallhagen, 1979).

Knowledge of the dominance over various functions of the right and left hemispheres and the symptomatology seen after right or left sided stroke assists the occupational therapist in differentiating the hemisphere and cerebral area affected (Booth, 1982; Tieton and Maloaf, 1982).

In the history and physical assessment, the therapist looks for unreported symptoms, normal patterns and other problems which may impact this condition. It is also necessary to determine whether any detected deficits were present before or only after the stroke. Factors which should be assessed in an acute stroke patient and which are used in prognosis are summarized below (adapted with own modifications from Howe, 1977; Weiner and Goetz, 1981):

- Skin: prone to breakdown, diminished sensation;
- Head and neck: trauma, headache, dizziness, seizure, photophobia, stiff neck, drainage from ears/nose, variety of cranial nerve deficits;
- Respiratory: ability to protect and clear airway;
- Cardiovascular: lying, sitting or bilateral blood pressure, heart disease;
- Gastrointestinal: note any nausea, vomiting, special diet, signs of ulcer, bowel patterns;
- Genitourinary: presence of infection, prostrate enlargement, urinary patterns, continence, changes in sexual function;
- Neurological: levels of consciousness, reality orientation, cognition, judgement, memory, emotions/behaviour, reality language;
- Movement: ability to carry out purposeful movements, co-ordination, flaccidity/spasticity, involuntary movements, reflexes (Babinski's present), gait, posture;
- Visual: two-point discrimination, stereognosis, joint position, figure writing;
- Hearing: attentiveness.

The following factors were identified from past studies as being possible contributors to stroke patient recovery. Thompson and Coleman (1987e,f,g) have used these factors in a questionnaire for a National Stroke Survey. This collection of factors was original and had not been used in any previous questionnaire:

1. Age. Older stroke patients generally have less chance of a good recovery or even survival;
2. Number of previous strokes. Good prognosis is generally considered to decrease with an increase in the number of stroke incidences;
3. Handedness. It is still unclear if left- or right-handedness is a predictor of stroke recovery but it can be useful in explaining recovery in terms of cerebral hemisphere dominance, especially with respect to loss of language which is normally associated with the left hemisphere;
4. Affected side. Again, this is linked with cerebral dominance of the individual; if he/she is right-handed and has a right-handed stroke, then he/she will face greater difficulties during recovery;
5. Complications. A number of complications (as detailed previously) are thought to impede stroke recovery. In particular, these are;
   arteriosclerosis, contracture, double vision, hemianopia, hypertension, left ventricular failure (LVF) and aphasia;
6. Conditions. A range of conditions may also affect recovery angina, diabetes, epilepsy, etc.;
7. Severity of stroke. The more severely affected the patient is by the stroke, the less chance he/she has of a good recovery;
8. Type of stroke. Generally, a non-ischaemic stroke is more dangerous than an ischaemic stroke since the former is associated with a cerebral aneurysm (a balloon-shaped swelling). If this ruptures blood can pour into the spaces of the brain to cause further loss of function. A blood clot, whether moving or stationary, is generally less of a risk and this is known as an aschaemic stroke;
9. Motivation. This is very important for the recovery of a stroke patient and is perhaps one of the more important aspects of the therapist's subjective evaluations. If the patient is highly motivated, he/she is usually observed to perform more successfully in therapeutic tasks and so, in turn, will aid his/her recovery;

10. Other factors. There are many other factors which are thought to be responsible for a stroke patient's recovery but none have been reliably identified as being actual predictors of recovery. These have included:
the sex of the patient, the type of therapy practised, the return of upper and lower limb function and the drugs administered during recovery.

Each of these factors was carefully considered and included in the survey questionnaire that was sent to occupational therapists around the country. The completed questionnaire provided valuable statistics for these stroke factors.

Past studies have also attempted to quantify some of these factors: e.g. by scoring videos of patient's performances in upper limb tasks (Turczynski, Hartje and Sturm, 1984); during re-education of affected upper limb muscles of CVA patients with expressive aphasia (Balliet, Levy and Blood, 1986; Bach-y-Rita, 1981); in comparing efficacy of conventional therapeutic exercises with an EMG biofeedback method (Chernikova, 1984). In the late 1980s these factors were used in computer programs towards the development of expert systems; however, this advance has been primitive in so far as it has involved only a feasibility study of a physician-developed expert system (Tuhrim and Reggia, 1986) and the use of microcomputers to support a database for stroke diagnosis (Banks, Caplan and Hier, 1983; Hier et al., 1986). Expert systems have also been used for the evaluation of abnormal locomotion arising from stroke (Dzierzanowski et al., 1985) and for computer-aided diagnosis (Fieschi et al., 1982) but it was not until 1985 that they were used for the prognosis of a stroke, albeit based on perceptual disabilities of stroke patients (McSherry and Fullerton, 1985).

About 25% of patients who fail to recover fully from stroke suffer one or more perceptual disorders (Adams and Hurwitz, 1983). The major perceptual disorders in stroke are: neglect, in which the hemiparetic patient tends to ignore his/her surroundings on the affected side of the body (see Figure 1.4 for clock-drawing task); disorder of spatial orientation, in which the patient has difficulty in appreciating relationships; and denial, in which the patient may even deny ownership of the weak limbs. Any combination of these disorders may occur. The prognostic significance in stroke of perceptual disorders has been widely recognized (Feigenson, McCarthy and Meese, 1977). In spite of the importance of these

19

Figure 1.4 Clock drawing – typical of a patient with neglect due to a lesion of the right hemisphere.

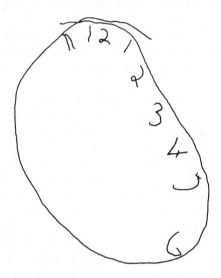

disorders, however, their diagnosis can present considerable difficulties due to differences in terminology, the lack of standardization of test methods and the frequent inability of stroke patients to comply with existing tests. In the Thompson and Coleman (1987e,f) research, patients were selected who did not present with such perceptual disabilities, but rather were absent in the usual proprioceptive capabilities (such as knowing where to and when a limb has moved) and suffered neuromuscular dysfunction (e.g., as shown by poor muscular reaction times, etc.).

They also addressed the subject of uncertainty raised by Speigelhalter and Knill-Jones (1984) who suggested that where uncertainty exists, it should be reliably quantified and justified to clinicians on the basis of extensive recorded experience. In accordance with past studies that used mathematical models to represent data (Smith, 1975; 1978) Bayesian Theory was considered and conditional probability formulae used to calculate the probabilities of occurrence of the various stroke factors used in the questionnaire and in earlier patient testing trials.

A National Stroke Survey

In the Thompson and Coleman (1987f) study, 100 occupational therapy departments were randomly selected from a cross-section of all the Regional Health Authorities in Great Britain using the *Hospital and Health Services Year Book* directory (Chapman, 1986). Letters were addressed to the head occupational therapist of each department who was asked to complete and return an enclosed two-part survey form. Part A asked the therapist to complete the section concerning their prognosis of each patient on two occasions separated by a three-week period. Part B (which asked for a detailed medical history) was to be completed for each patient once only. The purpose of this procedure was so that a comparison could be made between patients, and also for each patient between week 1 and week 3 — hence determining whether or not the therapist's prognosis had changed.

Factors considered to be important in determining an overall picture of the stroke patient were gathered from a number of sources (Young and Reid, 1972; Sødring, 1980a; 1980b; Rose and Capildeo, 1981; Hart, 1983; Pinelli, 1984; Spiegelhalter and Knill-Jones, 1984; Goetter, 1986; Hier et al., 1986; Tuhrim and Reggia, 1986); and discussion with members of the treatment team who were drawn from the medical and paramedical professions also occurred. The factors were phrased concisely and formed the questionnaire of the survey.

On examination of each therapist's comments regarding their prognosis, data were separated into two groups: out of the 94 patients detailed, 45 were given a poor prognosis on the second occasion (i.e. week 3) and 49 were given a good prognosis. Criteria used to determine poor and good prognosis were as follows:

The term poor prognosis was used when the therapist's comments stated that the patient was making very slow progress in therapeutic tasks; had poor return of function generally; was unable to cope with activities of daily living (ADL); was unable to walk (with or without assistance); and had deteriorated (or did not exhibit improvement) in health and/or progress from week 1.

The term good prognosis was used when the therapist's comments stated that the patient was making good progress in therapeutic tasks; had good return of function generally;

21

was able to cope with ADL; was now able to walk (with or without assistance); and had improved in health and/or progressed from week 1.

There were 47.87% patients with a poor prognosis and 52.13% with a good prognosis. The frequency of occurrence was found for each factor on the survey form by totalling each occurrence (in each stroke group, poor or good prognosis) and dividing by the total number of patients in each of the two prognosis groups. This was then expressed as a percentage. Thus, for example, the number of left-sided stroke patients with a poor prognosis was $4/45=8.89\%$, as compared with $17/49$ in the good prognosis group, which is 34.69%. These findings are shown in Tables 1.3 and 1.4.

As the sample size was limited to the number of replies, there was insufficient data to provide statistically meaningful information for some of the factors used on the survey form. Such was the case for the age of the patient. In this instance the age range of 19–86 years was divided into four groups; 19–35 years, 36–52 years, 53–69 years, 70–86 years and percentage frequencies were calculated for each age range rather than finding the frequency for each age. Similarly, instead of presenting frequencies for each week post-stroke, four ranges were selected that were consistent with suggested data collection periods of past studies. These were: 4–16 weeks, 17–29 weeks, 30–42 weeks and 43–55 weeks.

Finally, in order to comprehensively represent the variety of drugs that were administered to patients of the survey, these drugs were categorized according to their major function. For example, Digoxin is administered for supraventricular arrhythmia, while Inderetic is essentially used for reducing hypertension. These arrangements of the data thus presented the findings in a more useful and meaningful way.

Outcome of stroke

An important area continually receiving considerable attention is the predictability of outcome following an acute stroke. The role of computer tomography (CT) is being explored, with a number of papers having been published concerning this topic (Miller and Miyamoto, 1979; Weisberg, 1979; Rosenberg and Koller, 1981). It would seem that an important determinant of the outcome after

Table 1.3
Percentage frequency of occurrence of factors found with 1. Poor prognosis; 2. Good prognosis; (from Thompson, 1987f), adjusted to 2 dec.pl.).

		% Frequency	
Stroke factor		Poor prognosis	Good prognosis
Age range	19–35 years	11.11	53.06
	36–52 "	11.11	16.33
	53–69 "	33.33	22.45
	70–86 "	44.44	8.16
Number of previous strokes	0	77.78	87.76
	1	11.11	12.24
	2	11.11	0.00
Handedness	left	2.22	4.08
	right	97.78	95.92
Affected side	left	8.89	34.69
	right	91.11	65.31
Most important complication	arteriosclerosis	8.89	0.00
	contracture	15.56	8.16
	double vision	15.56	0.00
	hemianopia	8.89	0.00
	hypertension	26.67	32.65
	left ventricular failure	8.89	0.00
	speech loss	15.56	0.00
	NONE	0.00	59.19
Most important condition	angina	33.33	18.37
	diabetes	11.11	10.20
	epilepsy	11.11	0.00
	NONE	44.45	71.43
Severity of stroke	mild	44.44	71.43
	severe	55.56	28.57
Type of stroke	ischaemic	15.56	36.73
	non-ischaemic	22.22	12.24
	unknown CVA	62.22	51.02

23

Table 1.4
Percentage frequency of occurrence of factors found with 1. Poor
prognosis; 2. Good prognosis; (from Thompson, 1987f), adjusted
to 2 dec.pl.). (continued)

		% Frequency	
Stroke factor		Poor prognosis	Good prognosis
Number of weeks	4–16 weeks	48.89	6.12
post-stroke	17–29 weeks	20.00	20.41
(on occasion of second	30–42 weeks	20.00	32.65
prognosis)	43–55 weeks	11.11	40.82
Motivation	high	4.44	63.27
	medium	0.00	26.53
	poor	95.56	10.20
Return of hand function	good	35.56	63.27
	poor	64.44	36.73
Return of leg function	good	46.67	87.76
(muscle tonus)	poor	53.33	12.24
Graded symptoms	1	6.67	12.24
	2	6.67	12.24
	3	6.67	38.78
	4	24.44	12.24
	5	44.44	12.24
	6	11.11	12.24
Sex	male	73.33	85.71
	female	26.67	14.29
Therapy practised	Bobath	60.00	87.75
	Rood	40.00	12.24
Major drugs administered for	angina (e.g. Nifedipine)	15.56	4.08
	anticoagulance (e.g. Heparin)	13.33	32.65
	arrhythmia (e.g. Atenolol)	11.11	12.24
	hypertension (e.g. Inderetic)	22.22	16.33

muscle spasm		
(e.g. Diazepam)	11.11	12.24
supraventricular		
arrhythmia		
(e.g. Digoxin)	8.89	2.04
(particularly		
arterial		
fibrillation)		
NONE	17.78	20.41

an acute stroke is the size of the lesion (Harrison and Dyken, 1983; Ross Russell, 1983). Lesion size, as measured by CT, correlates with functional outcome (Hay et al., 1984) but this does not necessarily prove that CT scanning is of prognostic value above clinical assessment. Allen (1984a) has described a prognostic discriminant function that predicts, from six clinical features only, the probability of a patient's functional outcome after a stroke. Results from the testing of large samples of patients seem to clearly indicate that CT scanning is necessary to make an accurate diagnosis after acute stroke (Allen, 1984b). As Allen (1984c) has suggested, this has prognostic relevance in so far as there is a difference in outcome between intracerebral haemorrhage and infarction. However, clinical assessment is usually sufficient to achieve a reasonably accurate prognosis, upon which the CT scanner can only improve marginally.

A variety of studies have been undertaken into the measurement of the factors affecting outcome following stroke, namely: age (Wade et al., 1984a); case fatality (Dennis and Warlow, 1987; Stevens and Amber, 1982); survival (Wade et al., 1984b); recurrence (Dennis and Warlow, 1987); disability (Heinemann et al., 1987) and psychological and social outcome (Lawrence and Christie, 1979; Isaacs, Neville and Rushford, 1976).

These are important factors to consider as they can be used to monitor the impact of disease on society, act as a basis for prognosis prediction and give researchers a baseline on which to continue their studies (Gresham, 1986). Gresham also suggests that a consistent methodological approach is required in stroke outcome studies to ensure that these three elements are rigorously addressed.

FURTHER READING

Aetiology

Bach-y-Rita, P. (1981) Brain plasticity as a basis for the development of rehabilitation procedures for hemiplegia, *Scand. J. Rehab. Med.*, **13**, 73–83.

Family involvement

Drummond, A.E.R. (1988) Stroke: The impact on the family, *Brit. J. Occupat. Ther.*, **51**, no. 6, 193–4.

Mykyta, L.J., Bowling, J.H., Nelson, D.A. and Lloyd, E.J. (1976) Caring for relatives of stroke patients, *Age and Ageing*, **5**, 87–90.

Incidence and risk factors

Dennis, M.S. and Warlow, C.P. (1987) Stroke – Incidence, risk factors and outcome, *Brit. J. Hosp. Med*, **3**, 194–8.

Goldberg, G. and Berger, G.G. (1988) Secondary prevention in stroke: A primary rehabilitation concern, *Arch. Phys. Med. Rehabil.*, **69**, 32–40.

Kannel, W.B. and Wolf, P.A. (1983) Epidemiology of cerebrovascular disease, in *Vascular Disease of the Central Nervous System* (ed. R.W. Ross Russell), 2nd edn., Churchill Livingstone, Edinburgh, pp. 1–24.

Memory

Tepperman, P.S., Sovic, R. and Devlin, H.T.M. (1986) Stroke rehabilitation: A problem orientated approach, *Stroke*, **80**, no. 8, (Postgraduate Medicine), 158–67.

Wade, D.T., Parker, V. and Hewer, R.L. (1986) Memory disturbances after stroke: Frequency and associated losses, *Int. Rehabil. Med.*, **8**, 65–8.

National Stroke Survey

Thompson, S.B.N. and Coleman, M.J. (1987) An investigation into stroke, *Ther. Week.*, **13**, no. 29, 7.

Thompson, S.B.N. and Coleman, M.J. (1988) Occupational therapists' prognoses of their patients: Findings of a British survey of stroke, *Int. J. Rehabilitation Res.*, **11**, no. 3, in press.

Neuroanatomy

Luciano, S.D., Vander, A.J. and Sherman, J.H. (1978) *Human Anatomy and Physiology: Structure and Function*, 2nd edn, McGraw-Hill.

Tortora, G.J. and Anagnostakos, N.P. (1987) *Principles of Anatomy and Physiology*, 5th edn, Harper and Row, chs 14, 15.

2

Assessment

OCCUPATIONAL THERAPY ASSESSMENT

Why do we assess?

It is important to address the reasons for assessment before moving forward into areas of treatment. How do we know which areas to encourage our patients to work on unless we know which areas are deficient? It is also important to clarify assessment as separate from treatment. So often we see assessment tests or procedures repeated as treatment activities with little or no reward to the patient. There is also the possibility that the patient will learn the assessment tasks, thereby invalidating the level of improvement seen.

There are two main reasons why we should carefully assess the patients in our care; firstly, to establish a baseline in order to measure improvement; and secondly, to enable decisions to be made with the patient regarding priority areas for treatment:

1. Establishing a baseline.
    Early assessment is the key to motivating patients towards recovery. If patients are able to see improvement measured against initial performance it will motivate them to progress further;
2. Establishing priorities.
    The patient's idea of priorities to be addressed may be different to the therapist's. For example, the therapist may think that dressing skills are of prime importance when the patient actually wishes to be independent in transfers to the commode even if it means remaining in night-wear.
    Therefore, it is crucial for the therapist to take the patient's views as paramount ensuring maximum motivation for the rehabilitation programme.

Where do we assess?

The three main places where the OT may assess the patient are:

1. Hospital ward.
   In the early stages of recovery from stroke the patient is most likely to be in hospital. The hospital ward therefore becomes the first venue for assessment. Here the initial interview and discussions involving the family can take place and rapport-building can commence. It is vital to create as private an environment as possible (for example, using a side room rather than remaining behind screens in the main ward). This ensures that the personal nature of the questions asked do not compromize the patient's privacy.

2. The occupational therapy department.
   As soon as the patient is well enough to attend the OT department (ie. cope with the journey and duration of the sessions, etc.) it is advantageous to remove the patient from the ward environment. In the OT department more specific and in-depth assessments can be carried out such as perceptual testing and communication skills. Similarly, specialized equipment such as computer-based assessment tools may be available in the OT department but not necessarily elsewhere.

3. The home.
   As far as the patient is concerned this is probably the most important place for an assessment. This assessment can take place in the initial stages of rehabilitation as a home visit carried out by the therapist alone. Here the therapist may take the opportunity to talk to the patient's carers. Another visit is usually done prior to discharge in order to assess the patient's level of function in the home environment. Alternatively, a home visit by an OT may be made following referral by the General Practitioner as a consequence of a mild stroke and where some minor problems have been identified.

When do we assess?

Assessment is considered by the therapist to be a continuous process. The therapist will continually be aware of changes in the patient's performance without necessarily carrying out formal assessments. However, in order to measure more specific improvements in all areas of treatment there are several occasions when formal assessment is required; for example, when the patient is first seen (initial interview). This may be followed by graded assessments in areas such as personal care activities, perception, domestic activities of daily living, employment and leisure activities.

What do we assess?

The three main areas for assessment are: the patient; the family; and the home. The most crucial of these is the patient, his or her ability to perform tasks of daily living and any deficient areas requiring attention. In this way the patient can be assisted to establish priorities.

The patient

Communication Work already carried out or in progress by the speech therapist should be monitored and reinforced during therapy sessions. It is essential for all therapists concerned to be consistent with commands and gestures especially if comprehension appears to be affected. Good communication is vital in rapport building: an essential process if results are to be forthcoming. If the patient's communication problems are expressive in nature, then picture-pointing boards are useful tools to try. Other methods which can be used are mime, written messages, demonstrations or sensory input via hands or parts of the body.

Communication can be assessed easily on first contact with the patient by requesting simple tasks to be performed; e.g. requesting identification of clothes and familiar objects (testing receptive and expressive skills); and requesting selection of specific items from a bedside locker (to test comprehension and receptive skills).

Common language deficits The area of the brain responsible for language and speech lies in the dominant hemisphere, namely the left hemisphere in right-handed people and in a large percentage of left-handed people. Dysphasia is one of the most common language problems seen in association with right hemiplegia but in a number of cases the plegia recovers fully leaving the patient with no apparent physical disability. In a few cases, dysphasia is associated with left hemiplegia. The nature and severity of the disorder depends upon the site and severity of the lesion.

Dysphasia may be regarded primarily as a disorder of language resulting from brain injury. It has been defined as 'a reduction of available language affecting all language modalities (i.e. comprehension of the spoken and written word and expression of spoken and written language) and it may or may not be accompanied by other specific perceptual or sensorimotor deficits compatable with brain damage'.

Dysphasia is usually considered in two forms: receptive dysphasia (the impairment of comprehension of language, both oral and written); and expressive dysphasia (disorder of the expression of language, both oral and written). Associated with dysphasia are the following terms:

1. Global dysphasia.
   A disorder which results in impairment of all language modalities; i.e. poor comprehension of the spoken and written word combined with poor expression of the language, oral and written;
2. Jargon dysphasia.
   (a) English jargon: the production of a string of English words uttered with conventional intonation patterns, but which do not obey rules of semantics or syntax and which make no sense. This type of speech has also been described as 'word salad';
   (b) Neologistic jargon: the production of a string of nonsense syllables, again uttered with normal intonation patterns;
3. Recurrent utterance.
   The continuous production of one word or phrase in response to different stimuli. The utterance may be used with different intonation patterns to convey varying emotions. For example, 'money, money'; 'Dee, Dee'; 'I think one, two'. Recurrent utterance should never be reinforced and attempts should be made to encourage the patient to produce a different response through the use of cueing (e.g. prompting the patient with the first letter or syllable of the word);
4. Paraphasias.
   (a) Literal paraphasia: the patient substitutes one or more sounds in a word but leaves more than half of the word correctly articulated. Literal paraphasic errors are produced in a fluent manner with no evidence of struggling behaviour, e.g. chair – 'tair', carpet – 'tarpet';

31

(b) Verbal paraphasia: the patient produces a word that is a recognizable word and is associated in some way with the target word. Once more, these words are produced in a fluent manner, e.g. chair – 'tabie';
5. Neologisms.
This term refers to the production of nonsense syllables which bear no resemblance to the target word;
6. Neologistic distortion.
In an effort to produce a target word, a word is uttered fluently but less than half of the word is correctly articulated, e.g. chair – 'chact';
7. Circumlocution.
In an effort to produce the target word, the patient talks round the word without being able to recall the appropriate word, e.g. 'I would like a – you know – one of those things – you know, you write with';
8. Perseveration.
The inability to inhibit a previous response when presented with a new stimulus;
9. Paralexic errors.
The production of words associated with the target word in oral reading;
10. Dysgraphia.
A disorder of writing;
11. Echolalia.
Imitation of the stimulus word, phrase or sentence in response to the stimulus.

Speech deficits
1. Articulatory dyspraxia.
This has been defined as the inability to produce voluntary movements of the articulators in the absence of paralysis. Dyspraxics are therefore able to chew and swallow normally and can produce all movements of the articulators involuntarily but are unable to produce these movements on demand. Dyspraxia may exist as an isolated disorder but it is more commonly seen in conjunction with dysphasia;
2. Dysarthria.
This is a disorder of articulation resulting from weakness or paralysis of the muscles of articulation. It affects the following aspects of speech production: articulation, resonance, voice quality, intonation and rhythm of speech. The following are

three main types of dysarthria that may be associated with stroke patients:

(a) lower motor neurone dysarthria: this type of dysarthria arises from a lesion of the lower motor neurone supplying the speech musculature. It results in a flaccid paralysis of the muscles. All types of movement are affected by the lesion, i.e. voluntary, involuntary and reflex. Speech characteristics:
   - voice: breathing quality;
   - poor breath control;
   - intonation monotonous;
   - hypernasality: i.e. excessive nasal resonance and nasal emission;
   - diminished or absent gag reflex;
   - weak or slurred articulation;
   - occasional vowel distortion;
   - excessive drooling;
   - difficulty chewing and swallowing;

(b) upper motor neurone dysarthria: lesion of the upper motor neurone results in a spastic weakness of the muscles of articulation. Speech characteristics:
   - voice: harsh quality (sometimes breathy pitch breaks);
   - poor breath control;
   - intonation monotonous;
   - reduced stress;
   - tongue movement is sluggish and movements tend to be laboured;
   - imprecision of consonental articulation;
   - some hypernasality;
   - difficulty in chewing and swallowing;
   - excessive drooling;

(c) cerebellar dysarthria: characteristically dysarthria only results from bilateral lesion of the cerebellum or the cerebellar connections with the brain stem. Speech characteristics:
   - voice: harsh quality, pitch breaks, excessive volume, voice tremor, habitual pitch abnormally high;
   - in-coordination of expiration and phonation;
   - monotonous intonation;
   - stress and rhythm deviant: scanning is of syllabic quality (i.e. equal stress being placed on each syllable).

Personal activities of daily living In the early stages of rehabilitation personal care tasks can be used as assessment tools. Communication and perception difficulties as well as general muscle weakness can clearly be identified during these activities. It is important, however, to identify whether the cause is perceptual or functional. The following table shows how simple everyday tasks can be used in the assessment process:

- Eating and Drinking

Task	Assessment
Picking up and manipulating cutlery	Grip strength, manual dexterity and level of return of function
Raising food or cup to mouth	Hand–eye–mouth co-ordination
Completing meal (without leaving half)	Recognition of body image; hemianopia
Finding cup placed on affected side	Hemianopia or neglect

- Toileting

Task	Assessment
Making request known	Aphasia, dysphasia or other speech problems
Stand, locate and walk to toilet	Hemiplegia, memory, mobility, walking gait and balance
Ability to manage clothes	Upper limb function; balance; dressing dyspraxia
Washing hands	Upper-limb function and neglect

- Washing and dressing

Task	Assessment
Washing face and body	Sitting balance, posture and neglect
Dressing upper half of body	Sitting to standing; comprehension of instructions or new techniques; ability to dress one-handed
Dressing lower half	Standing balance; manipulation of affected limbs

- Grooming

Task	Assessment
Shaving (men only!)	Sensory loss; hemianopia if using mirror; neglect
Brushing hair/teeth	Neglect or body image recognition

- Bathing

Task	Assessment
Getting in and out of the bath	Advanced mobility; balance; control of limbs; comprehension of safety aspects; heat/cold discrimination

Physical function The relationship between the physiotherapist and occupational therapist is of vital importance. Once an appropriate treatment approach has been identified all members of the team must use the same approach. Repetition of detailed physical

35

function assessment is unnecessary as well as being tiring and frustrating for the patient. Functional limitations such as spasticity can be noted during dressing assessment or other daily living activities. Close liaison with the physiotherapist will enable a complementary regime of activities to be established. Examples of occupational therapy and physiotherapy assessment charts can be seen later in this chapter.

Sensory function Loss of limb sensation affects voluntary movement in a number of ways with both exteroceptive and proprioceptive loss;

1. Exteroceptive loss.
   Lack of recognition by touch of shape, bulk and texture (otherwise known as asteriognosis). This is evident if the patient is unable to describe a common object held in the affected hand, e.g. a key. Localization of touch can be assessed by touching and asking the patient to point to the place where he/she was touched (both unaffected and affected sides should be tested);
2. Proprioceptive loss.
   Lack of sense of joint position. The patient is asked to catch hold of the thumb of the affected hand, first with eyes open and then shut.

Perception Another major area of work for occupational therapists is the assessment and treatment of perceptual problems. Edmans and Lincoln (1987) investigated the frequency of perceptual deficits after stroke. They found that perceptual problems were common in both left and right hemiplegic patients, where it was previously thought that patients with visual-perception disorders had predominantly right hemisphere lesions (i.e. left hemiplegics).

The four main areas of perceptual assessment are:

1. Body image/body schema.
   This is an appreciation of one's self within the environment. It can be seen when the patient attends to events and objects on the unaffected side only and yet when asked is aware of the other side as well. Examples of loss of body image include eating from only one half of the plate and washing and dressing the unaffected side only. However, this is not to be confused with hemianopia, which is the loss of

half of the visual field and is easily compensated for by head and eye movements. Most patients have good insight but a few do show separation from reality. Extreme cases tend to be right (non-dominant) hemiplegics but are most frequently left hemiplegics with parietal lobe damage. The patient may refuse to acknowledge that the arm is weak. This is known as anosognosia. Lack of awareness of self may result in denial of ownership of affected limbs. The patient may neglect the weak limb in spite of good motor and sensory recovery, requiring constant reminders to prevent damage.

2. Spatial relationships.
   This is where the patient has difficulty perceiving the position of two or more objects in relation to her-himself or each other, for example, when threading beads onto a string, the patient does not understand the relationships of beads to beads or beads to string. Further problems may include loss of ability to comprehend the relationship of objects in space due to lack of conception of three dimensions. The patient may collide with objects he/she can see (e.g. door frame) or may not be able to judge distances between objects. The patient may also have difficulty with subtle variations in form and so, for example, may confuse a box of tissues with a book. Interpretation of concepts such as in/out, up/down, in front/behind may also be affected.

3. Apraxia.
   This is when the patient cannot perform previously learnt skills even though comprehension, motor power, co-ordination and sensation are intact, e.g. events may be performed out of sequence (such as brushing teeth and then putting toothpaste on the brush); or not being able to use an item such as a hairbrush or pen for its proper use.

4. Agnosia.
   This is the lack of recognition of familiar objects perceived by the senses; i.e. visual, tactile, proprioceptive or auditory. An example of this could be where the patient fails to recognize objects even though visual ability and recognition of objects by touch are intact. Patients may fail to recognize their relatives, etc. They may also have the inability to recognize objects or forms by handling, even though tactile, thermal and proprioceptive functions are intact. This is known as astereognosis.

Domestic activities of daily living It is important to identify the patient's previous role in relation to domestic activities and the running of the home. A single person is likely to have all previous domestic tasks to return to but either partner in a couple may have taken certain responsibilities at home. The patient's partner may find themselves dealing with new areas such as housework or budgeting and finance. Assessment of domestic tasks should be done according to the patient's future needs when he/she is at home:

1. home management: including payment of bills, general finances, comprehension of money value, etc.;
2. shopping: frequency of trips and amount of help available;
3. cooking: types of meals eaten and previous skills used;
4. general housework and laundry: assessment of tasks previously undertaken at home and amount of help available.

The family

In the event of a stroke affecting a member of a family, the family's needs, fears and anxieties of the situation should be addressed as well as the needs of the patient. Hopefully, the family members will be closely involved with the rehabilitation and their co-operation will be gratefully received by all staff. Understanding the illness and associated problems is usually the first hurdle to help family members overcome by providing information at a suitable level and by answering questions appropriately. Any personality changes in the patient may be particularly difficult for the family to understand and they will need encouragement whilst recovery continues. The previous role of the patient should be identified and this may only be possible by asking the relatives questions about the general mood swings and participation in the family and community before the stroke onset. This will give some indication as to the level of recovery expected by the patient's family and their hopes for the patient's complete return to normal functioning. Partners, relatives or closely-connected friends involved in the set-up may find it useful to be in contact with a support group or social worker early on for support and advice outside the main hospital environment (Mykyta *et al.*, 1976). Documentation is sparse on the effects on the family as most literature concentrates on the stroke victim rather than others affected indirectly (Drummond, 1988; Thames and McNeil, 1987).

The home

A home-visit assessment may be carried out by the occupational therapist at any stage in the rehabilitation process. In the early stages the therapist may visit the home alone to see the partner, assess family members' reactions to the stroke patient and the general dynamics relating to the thought of the patient returning home. Later, the therapist will visit with the patient to assess the physical suitability of the home and facilities according to the amount of return of functional capabilities. Where mobility is reduced, particular areas for concern will include access to the house itself and use of the stairs. In some cases, where the patient uses a wheelchair, adaptations to provide suitable accessible facilities may be required.

In the later stages of rehabilitation, the patient will need to begin to look towards returning home and employment or alternative occupation. A work assessment may be done, in which case liaison with the employers would help the OT identify the requirements of the job in order to simulate them in the OT department. In cases where it becomes obvious that the previous tasks cannot be carried out, the Disablement Resettlement Officer may be invited to set-up alternative training opportunities. If no future employment is expected, advice regarding suitable leisure and social activities may be of assistance to the patient and to the family.

ASSESSMENT TESTS

A number of tests have been developed in an attempt to standardize the approach to the assessment of stroke patients (examples of assessment tests are described later). Some have been received with a degree of hesitancy as they can be lengthy to complete and limited in nature. Similarly, as each patient is an individual and does not necessarily fit into a standard model, some therapists prefer to use an open chart with space for comments only. However, with the increasing need for research into outcome and prognosis, some standard method of measuring and recording deficit and progress is essential. The data collected is also useful as a means of guiding the therapist towards implementing an appropriate treatment programme. Two examples of different sets of tests are:

1. The Chessington OT Neurological Assessment Battery (COTNAB).

   This has been developed by the staff of the Joint Services Medical Unit (RAF Chessington) and the Wolfson Medical Rehabilitation Centre (Atkinson Morley Hospital, London SW20). It is published by Nottingham Rehab. Limited. The assessment consists of twelve separate tests within four broad functional areas:
   (a) Visual perception
       – overlapping figures;
       – hidden figures;
       – sequencing;
   (b) Constructional ability
       – 2D construction;
       – 3D construction;
       – block printing;
   (c) Sensory-motor ability
       – stereognosis and tactile discrimination;
       – dexterity;
       – co-ordination;
   (d) Ability to follow instructions
       – written instruction;
       – visual instructions;
       – spoken instructions.

   For each test measures are obtained for ability to complete the task and the time taken, which are combined to provide a measure of overall performance. These tests, which are summarized later, do not aim to identify specific organic or psychological deficits but are intended to be standardized assessments of areas of functional ability related to the practise of occupational therapy. The assessment has been standardized on a population of 150 people unaffected by stroke within each of three age groups. Stroke patient scores on each test are then compared with these results for their age group in terms of ability, time and overall performance. The package includes the details of the tests and a therapists' note section for each test showing common errors, observed difficulties and possible explanations. A separate Treatment Resource File includes an introduction to the treatment of the neurological patient, suggested treatment activities for each of the four areas of assessment, a further section on group

Table 2.1
Description of individual COTNAB tests

Test	Description	Aims to assess
Visual perception		
Overlapping figures	Identification of shapes from a complex design	Form constancy
Hidden figures	Tracing around shapes within a design	Figure-ground discrimination
Sequencing	Placing sets of cards in their logical order	Logical sequencing
Constructional ability		
2–D Construction	Paper and pencil work mainly drawings	Constructional work in 2–D
3–D Construction	Reproductions of a 3–D model with replica blocks	Constructional work in 3–D
Block printing	Copying designs using printing blocks	More complex constructional work

treatment activities, an illustrative case example and reference material. For a description of the individual COTNAB tests, see Tables 2.1 and 2.2.

2. Tests for identification of disability in stroke patients.
    Bernard Isaacs (1971) compiled a series of twenty tests in response to his own frustration in assessing the perceptual and cognitive problems of his stroke patients. He instigated their use on one of his stroke wards and found them to be helpful in highlighting the areas in which patients were experiencing difficulty. He was then able to classify the results in terms of the major disability shown in the patients (table 2.3). Eight of the twenty tests are shown in Figures 2.1 to 2.10 as they are most relevant and familiar to occupational therapists working with stroke patients.

Table 2.2
Description of individual COTNAB tests (continued)

Test	Description	Aims to assess
Sensory-motor ability		
Stereognosis and tactile discrimination	Naming common objects and textures by touch	Sensory discrimination
Dexterity	Moving coloured discs on a large board	Speed and accuracy of dexterity
Co-ordination	Placing a pointer in a series of graded holes	Hand-eye co-ordination
Ability to follow instructions		
Written instructions	Making a coat hanger on a standard jig	Ability to follow written instructions
Visual instructions	Constructing a metal assembly from a series of photographs	Ability to follow visual instructions
Spoken instructions	Choosing 12 action cards to represent a story	Ability to follow verbal instructions and memory

ASSESSMENT CHARTS

An assessment chart should be an accurate, clear and concise record of the areas assessed by the therapist. It should be easy to understand, without the possibility of mis-interpretation by the chart users. It should provide a record of achievement for the patient and other disciplines and should cover all activities undertaken. Three examples (Figures 2.11–2.13) show the varying degree of depth and different methods of rating.

Figure 2.11 shows a general neurological and functional assessment chart in the form of a record sheet where comments are made by the therapist about each of the areas shown. This allows the therapist to have complete freedom to express their findings and concerns but it is difficult to ensure consistency of approach.

Figure 2.12 shows an assessment chart as described by

Table 2.3
Outcome of treatment of 115 stroke cases classified by type of disability (from Isaacs 1971)

	Type of disability				
	Motor	Communication	Perceptual	Cognitive	All strokes
Outcome of stay in stroke ward					
Discharged	16	18	19	9	62
Died	3	16	4	4	27
Transferred to long stay	4	9	8	5	26
Total	23	43	31	18	115
Outcome one year after onset					
At home	10	15	16	8	49
In hospital	5	9	6	2	22
Dead (Not yet	7	18	8	8	41
one year after onset)	1	1	1	0	3
Total	23	43	31	18	115

Karen Sødring (1980). This chart is more specific as it includes a rating system for each area assessed. This ensures consistency amongst therapists using this method.

Figure 2.13 shows a more typical occupational therapy chart particularly detailed to cover all activities of daily living broken down into component parts. Also included are the perceptual and cognitive areas, some of which may have been assessed using methods described earlier.

ROLE OF COMPUTERS IN ASSESSMENT PROCEDURES

The ability of computers to store and manipulate large amounts of data make them invaluable tools to the occupational therapist when assessing stroke patients. Studies carried out by Smith (1978) showed that computers can provide useful statistics for conditions such as stroke and myocardial infarction and indeed for

43

Figure 2.1 Orientation.

ORIENTATION

Object: To test memory and awareness of environment

Exclusions: Deaf; aphasia.

Materials: None.

Method: Examiner asks the following questions in order:

1. What is your name?;
2. What is your address?;
3. What day is it?;
4. What month is it?;
5. What year is it?;
6. What time is it?;
7. Where are you just now?;
8. How long have you been here?;
9. When is your birthday?;
10. Who am I?

Notes:

Q4. If test is given on first three days of month, allow previous month;

Q5. If test is given in January allow previous year;

Q6. Allow subject to consult clock; otherwise allow error of up to two hours;

Q7. Allow: 'in a hospital';

Q8. Allow up to 50% error;

Q10. Allow: 'the doctor';

Time: Less than 5 minutes.

Score: Score 1 for each correct answer. Score 0 for incorrect or no answer. (No half scores.)

Interpretation:
Correctly-oriented patients make less than three errors.

Figure 2.2 Digit reversal.

DIGIT REVERSAL

Object: To test short-term memory and mental flexibility

Exclusions: Deaf; aphasia.

Materials: None.

Method: Examiner says to subject:

'I am going to test your memory. I want you to remember this number . . . 729'.

'Can you repeat the number?'
If subject fails the test is stopped. If subject succeeds, examiner says:
'Now can you say that backwards?'

If subject succeeds proceed to four-digit number, etc. Use 2836; 41925.

Time: Less than one minute.

Score: Number of digits that subject is able to reverse.

Interpretation:
a. Failure to reverse 3 digits implies severe short-term memory loss;
b. Ability to reverse 4 digits implies good short-term memory.

Figure 2.3 Read the newspaper.

READ THE NEWSPAPER

Object: *To identify alexia, agnosia, neglect of left half of space*

Exclusions: Visual impairment from peripheral causes.

Materials: Newspaper.

Method: Examiner first checks that subject's eyesight is all right and that he is wearing suitable spectacles. He then gives paper to subject and asks him to read a headline. If this is correctly performed subject is then asked to read a short paragraph in large print and to summarize it. If headline is not read properly subject is asked to read the name of the newspaper, and if he still fails he is asked to point to prominent words in headline. If he still fails he is given instructions in writing, e.g. POINT TO THE WORD 'DAILY'.

Time: Less than one minute.

Score: No score.

Interpretation:

a. Patients with expressive aphasia who have no alexia correctly identify words on verbal or written instructions;

b. Patients with agnosia dismiss test without attempting it, or with excuses;

c. Patients with neglect of e.g. left half of space omit a word or words on left half of headline, and one or more words at beginning of every line of text without apparent perplexity. They may even begin in the middle of a word;

d. Patients with mental impairment are unable to summarize content of paragraph.

Figure 2.4 Picture identification.

PICTURE IDENTIFICATION

Object: *To test for visual agnosia, neglect of left half of space, abstract thought*

Exclusions: Peripheral visual impairment.

Materials: Newspaper (or specially mounted photograph).

Method: Subject is shown a suitable picture and asked: 'What do you see?' Picture should have two or more clearly identifiable persons or objects in it, and not too much detail. A photograph of a bride and groom is ideal. If subject cannot identify picture examiner asks:
'Is there a man in it?'
'Point to the man.'
'Is there anyone else?'
'Is there a woman?'
'Point to the woman.'
'What is the woman wearing?' etc.

Time: Less than one minute.

Score: No score.

Interpretation:

a. Patients with visual agnosia fail completely;

b. Patients with neglect of left half of space fail to identify figures in left half of picture;

c. Patients with loss of abstract thought fail to provide general interpretation of picture, e.g. call a bride a 'woman' or may misidentify picture on basis of misinterpretation of one detail, e.g. bride is described as a nurse.

Figure 2.5 Object identification.

OBJECT IDENTIFICATION

Object: To test for visual agnosia, perception of colour, size, texture, function: also language disturbances, especially name–finding; also tactile agnosia (astereognosia)

Exclusions: Blind; aphasia.

Materials: Common objects found in ward, e.g. bowl of fruit, bottle of mineral water, tumbler, comb, cosmetics, bed linen, etc.

Method: Examiner holds up object and asks:
'What is this?'
'What colour is it?'
'What do you do with it?'
'Show me what you do with it'.
If subject fails with any object, e.g. an apple, examiner places it in front of subject, together with one, then more than one dissimilar object, e.g. comb, and then says:
'Pick up the apple'.
'Pick up the red one'.
'Pick up the big one'.
'Pick up the round one'.
'Pick up the one you eat'. etc.
Examiner then tests the subject's ability to identify.

Score: No score.
Interpretation Test identifies:
a. Pure word finding difficulty (patient unable to name object but knows its function and its properties);
b. Loss of awareness of function of object (visual agnosia);
c. Loss of ability to identify it by touch (tactile agnosia).

---

any number of chronic diseases (Hill and Smith, 1974; Smith, 1975). The advantages of creating chronic disease data banks (Starmer, Rosati and McNeer, 1974a; Beilin *et al.*, 1974) and using computers as diagnostic and treatment planning aids (Starmer, Rosati and McNeer, 1974b; Coe *et al.*, 1975) are well documented. All that is needed is suitable hardware and software. If occupational therapists have access to computers with suitable, easy-to-use database enquiry programs, then computer models can help the therapist make more efficient and effective assessments and prognoses. Other areas of computer application have included the analysis of electroencephalograms (EEGs) from

Figure 2.6 Draw a man (see Figure 2.7).

DRAW A MAN

Classify: Normal; or evidence abnormality (specify).

Object: *To observe conceptualization and execution*

Exclusions: Sensory aphasia (incomprehension of instructions); blindness.

Materials: Felt-tip pen, paper.

Method: Examiner says to subject: 'Draw a little man for me on this piece of paper'. If subject fails to draw, examiner draws a man and says: 'Now you copy that'. NB — Give subject a large, plain sheet of paper.
Time: Less than one minute.
Score: Classify — Normal; or evidence of abnormality (specify).

Interpretation:

a. Note subject's attitude to test–enthusiasm or avoidance (e.g. 'I can't draw'; 'I need my spectacles', etc.);

b. In right hemiplegics make due allowance for difficulty in left-handed drawing, but subject often uses this as an excuse for not drawing, and this is not valid;

c. Note position of drawing on page: patients with neglect of left half of space place drawing on right half of page;

d. Note size of drawing; demented patients tend to make a very small drawing;

e. Note sophistication of drawing: this seems to reflect pre-morbid intellectual level;

f. Note relationship of body parts to one another: disrupted in cases of agnosia;

g. Omission of left half of drawing (e.g. representation of right arm or right leg) — characteristic of severe neglect of left hand of space;

h. Note evidence of inability to draw coherently, due to apraxia: and of repetitive scribbling, due to perseveration.

---

stroke patients (Cohen, Bravo-Fernandez and Sances, 1976a,b) and a microcomputer-based data handling and data retrieval system for stroke assessment (Thompson, 1987b).

Quantitative assessments using computer-compatible functional profiles of stroke have also been developed (Feigenson *et al.*, 1979). It is perhaps fruitful to consider one such study which focused on the team approach to patient care, which is a major factor in allowing so many patients to resume a reasonably independent existence at home. Experience with this approach led Feigenson and colleagues (1979) to recognize the need for a short yet comprehensive time-oriented profile to evaluate and document

Figure 2.7 The responses of patients with different disabilities to the request 'draw a man'. (From Isaacs, 1971.)

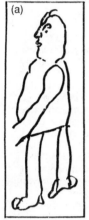

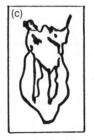
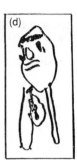

(a) Minimal brain damage.
(b) Gross generalised brain damage.
(c) Right hemiplegia and aphosia.
(d) Left hemiplegia and agnosia.
(e) Left hemiplegia with neglect of left half of space.
(f) Left hemiplegia; visual agnosia.

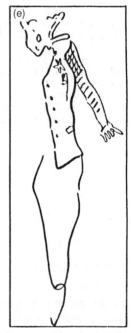
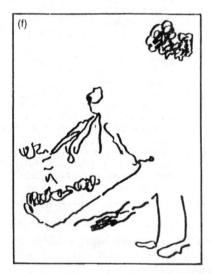

all phases of patient function. The Burke Stroke Time-Oriented Profile (BUSTOP) was developed and included the following needs:

1. An approach that stressed function rather than dysfunction;
2. Prospective measurements of progress during the rehabilitation phase of stroke;
3. Development of a computer-compatible quantitative measurement of the patient's overall status over time which

Figure 2.8 Draw a house, draw a clock (see Figure 2.9).

DRAW A HOUSE, DRAW A CLOCK

Object: *To test concept retention and execution and to test for neglect of half of space*

Exclusions: Blind, sensory aphasia.

Materials· Paper and felt-tip pen.

Method: Examiner says to subject:
1. 'I want you to draw a house';
2. 'I want you to draw a clock face with the numbers on it'.
Separate sheet of clean paper provided for each drawing. If subject fails examiner makes a simple drawing on his own and asks subject to copy it.

Time: One minute.

Score: Score as normal or impaired, specifying impairment.

Interpretation:
House:
a. Lack of perspective and lack of detail indicate low pre-morbid mentality or pathological brain damage;
b. Misplacement of features, e.g. windows, or chimney detached from remainder of house, indicates agnosia;
c. Drawing executed in interrupted lines may be due to apraxia;
Clock:
a. Numbers not all contained within clock face — general brain damage;
b. Numbers on left side omitted — neglect of left half of space.

---

would give information necessary for a time-oriented stroke database system;

4. Evaluation of the effectiveness of different therapeutic programmes with a well defined and standardized assessment of outcome;

5. An effort to minimize record keeping and maximize information while still maintaining a simple way to visualize patient progress from initial evaluation through discharge and follow-up;

6. Establishment of a standard method of charting that would allow for objective medical audit and provide information about the cost and effectiveness of medical care;

7. Determination of whether or not there are significant differences in a patient's performance in various disciplines and if so, to document these differences.

Prior to developing this particular profile, some pre-existing rating scales were reviewed. The Kenny Self-Care Evaluation (Iverson *et al.*, 1979) was considered too lengthy and stressed function alone without considering influencing factors such as confusion or depression. The PULSES index (Moskowitz and McCann, 1967) covered all aspects of patient performance but was

Figure 2.9 The responses of patients with different disabilities to the request 'draw a house and draw a clock'. (From Isaacs, 1971.)

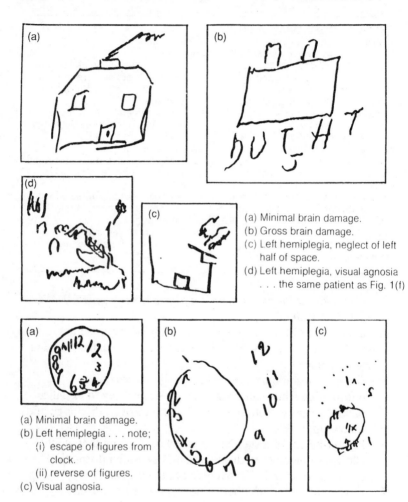

(a) Minimal brain damage.
(b) Gross brain damage.
(c) Left hemiplegia, neglect of left half of space.
(d) Left hemiplegia, visual agnosia . . . the same patient as Fig. 1(f)

(a) Minimal brain damage.
(b) Left hemiplegia . . . note;
　(i) escape of figures from clock.
　(ii) reverse of figures.
(c) Visual agnosia.

apparently too general for the experimental setting. The Barthel Index (Mahoney and Barthel, 1965) and the ADL−2 Profile used by the Burke Rehabilitation Center Day Hospital were less inclusive than PULSES and the categories were again rated as being too general.

Objective methods for scoring each area of function using the BUSTOP score sheets were developed and standardized. Computer-generated graphic displays of the data gathered on a

Figure 2.10 Two pen test.

TWO PEN

Object: *To demonstrate neglect of one half of space.*

Exclusions: Blind, sensory aphasia.

Materials: Two ball point pens or two pencils or similar objects of contrasting colours, e.g. one red and one blue.

Method: Examiner holds up two pens vertically about 12 inches in front of plane of patient's eyes, one pen in each hand, and separated from each other by about 12 inches. He asks: 'What do you see?' If subject says 'Two pens' examiner asks: 'What colour are they?' If subject answers correctly test is completed. If subject answers 'A pen', examiner asks: 'What colour is it?' and notes answer. Examiner then interchanges positions of pens in front of patient and asks subject again 'What do you see?' (A pen.) 'What colour is it?' Examiner then repeats test, holding two pens one inch apart.

Time: Less than one minute.

Score: Score as No/Mild/Severe neglect of left/right half of space.

Interpretation:

a. Patient with neglect of, e.g. left half of space sees only pen in right visual field;

b. Patient with hemianopia sees both pens when they are interchanged in front of his eyes, because he follows the pen into the blind half of his visual field;

c. In severe neglect only one pen is seen even when pens are less than one inch apart, and even when they are interchanged in front of subject's eyes.

---

sample patient were produced. Each graph illustrated progress over time as an average response of all raters in each of the major categories on a weekly basis. BUSTOP was used for four years and proved valuable in the rehabilitation setting, fulfilling most of the goals that led to its development. However, because patients react differently when treated by different members of the stroke team, ratings by nurses, physiotherapists and occupational therapists often differed. Analysis of the reasons for this variability in observed performance can often lead to improved therapeutic technique.

It must be said that time-oriented profiles measuring neurological deficit, ability to communicate and ability to perform cognitive and perceptual tasks must be added to any functional profile in order to create a meaningful, comprehensive stroke database system. As with many computer-based techniques that assist in assessing a neurological condition, while the objectiveness of the approach is meritable, the conclusions are often specific to the task or to the experimental setting. Therefore, caution must be exercised in any analysis of the results obtained under these conditions. In the past, a number of different methods have been used to assess motor behaviour in patients (Brunnström, 1962; 1970; Perry, 1967; Bobath, 1971; 1977; 1985; Danniels and Worthington, 1972; Hoskins and Squires, 1973) including the detailed monitoring of muscle movement for the verification of functional anatomies (Arsenault and Chapman, 1974), and a time-oriented profile for stroke patients (Feigenson *et al.*, 1979).

Some assessment procedures that have involved collection of large quantities of information have made use of information technology (Smith, 1978); and a survey conducted at the beginning of the 1980s revealed that some 69% of 301 psychophysiological laboratories in the United States were now equipped with computers for such usage (Buzzi and Battig, 1983). Computers are also increasingly being used for the collection of clinical data in Great Britain, with advancements that have included the use of a minicomputer to produce three-dimensional graphics of arteries of the heart, which are being used by Dr. Alan Colchester (Senior Registrar in neurology at St. George's Hospital and Atkinson Morley's Hospital, Wimbledon) and Mr. David Hawkes (Principal Physicist at St George's Hospital Department of Medical Physics) to help reduce coronary and stroke mortality (Bolton, 1985).

A computerized system for simultaneously recording and analysing several bioelectrical signals has also been developed (Buzzi and Battig, 1983). This system collected data from a series of incoming signals that included: electrocardiogram, respiration, skin conductance, electromyogram (EMG), plethysmogram, pulse transmission time (PTT) and EEG. The raw values for all these bioelectrical signals, except EMG and PTT, were collected on magnetic tape. How this system differed from previous studies was that the signals were detected by the appropriate devices and then read into a minicomputer for analysis. Similar research, using a more sophisticated method, samples one of these signals using an electromyograph-microcomputer link so that the complete measurement process of detection and interpretation is automatic (Thompson, 1987b,e,f).

Other computerized approaches to assessment and prognosis of neurological deficiencies such as stroke have been extremely complicated; for example, the use of computerized tomography as a prognostic tool (Hertann *et al.*, 1984). These approaches have also often demonstrated and concluded that sequential functional assessments, such as those used in the Thompson, Coleman and Yates (1986) study and in the Thompson (1987f) research, are in fact of more prognostic value. Support for this conclusion has been shown on a number of occasions (Fugl-Meyer *et al.*, 1975; An, Chao and Asken, 1980; De Souza, Langton-Hewer and Miller, 1980; Visser and Aanen, 1981; Logigian *et al.*, 1983; Pinelli, 1984).

The versatility of microcomputers has been widely recognized by researchers and clinicians and their direct role in a number of therapeutic settings has been documented, e.g. as a computer-aided diagnosis and assessment tool (Fieschi *et al.*, 1982; Allen, 1984b; Hier *et al.*, 1986); as a source of reference in the form of databases (Banks, Caplan and Hier, 1983) and in the measurement of functional capabilities of patients (Thompson, 1985a; Thompson and Coleman, 1987a,c). However, it is the direct use of microcomputers that is most exciting in terms of technological progress (Ediss and Grove, 1983; Hume, 1984). Microcomputer technology has reduced the time spent during assessments of motor, perceptual and memory function – the capabilities enable fast and accurate measurements to be made with a reduction in human error as machines can often replicate procedures more consistently than therapists or clinicians in some settings. Such was the case in the Thompson and Coleman (1987a,c) studies where an interactive system (i.e. involving communication between the therapist, user and the computer) enabled accurate and reliable measurements to be made of the electrical discharge from the leg muscles of stroke patients in order to assess their degree of motor and perceptual function. The microcomputer used could also store large amounts of data which was retrieved for later reference and comparisons. Banks, Caplan and Hier (1983) acknowledged the use of microcomputers for storing patient data and later Hier *et al.* (1986) used patient databases to build an expert system for the diagnosis of stroke.

Microcomputers are becoming increasingly important not only as a means of storage and for the fast retrieval of patient assessment data but also for direct measurements during functional assessments, especially for memory function (Skilbeck, 1984). McSherry and Fullerton (1985) recognized this use and developed an assessment schedule for perceptual neglect and investigated the possibilities of developing an expert system for the prognosis of stroke – a topic that has been extensively researched in a number of studies (Thompson, 1987a; Thompson and Coleman, 1987a,b,c).

Figure 2.11 Example of physiotherapy chart.

NAME:	DATE:
INDEX NO:	

MOTOR AND SENSORY ASSESSMENT
POSTURE
LYING
SITTING
STANDING

TONE
LEGS
ARMS
TRUNK

LEGS
JOINT RANGES
MOVEMENTS

ARMS
JOINT RANGES
MOVEMENTS

TRUNK
JOINT RANGES
MOVEMENTS

PROPRIOCEPTION
ARMS
LEGS

PINPRICK
ARMS
LEGS

STEREOGNOSIS

OTHER PROBLEMS	SOCIAL SITUATION

OTHER PROBLEMS
1. FACE;
2. ORIENTATION;
3. MOOD;
4. COMMUNICATION;
5. COMPREHENSION;
6. PERCEPTION;
7. INATTENTION;
8. DYSPRAXIA;
9. HEMIANOPIA;
10. CONTINENCE;
11. SWALLOWING;
12. SPEECH;
13. HEARING;
14. OTHER.

SOCIAL SITUATION

DRUGS

BALANCE AND WEIGHT-BEARING

SITTING – STATIC
        – DYNAMIC

STANDING – STATIC
        -- DYNAMIC

ROLLING

TO RIGHT
TO LEFT

SITTING TO STANDING

TRANSFERS

TO RIGHT
TO LEFT

WALKING GAIT

UP FROM FLOOR

STAIRS

GENERAL MOBILITY

WHEELCHAIR ETC.
INDOOR/OUTDOOR

Figure 2.12 Example of assessment chart. (from Sødring, 1980).

NUMERICAL EVALUATION:

− = Unable to perform the test;

0 = Cannot perform passive movement through full range of motion;

1 = Can perform passive movement through full range of motion, but cannot hold the position in the inner range without help;

2 = Can hold position — test position — alone;

3 = Can perform the test actively without help, but in an abnormal way (record that which is wrong, in synergy etc);

4 = Can perform the test in a normal way, but the quality of the performance is not completely normal (speed, precision);

5 = Normal active movement and performance.

Balance reactions are recorded by + or −

NAME:

AGE:

DATE OF ONSET:

SIDE:

SENSATION:

a) touch;

b) pain;

c) position sense.

POSTURAL TONE:

a) at rest;

b) associated reactions.

SUPINE

Tested by							
Date							
Leg	Score	Remarks	Score	Remarks	Score	Remarks	Score	Remarks
1. Sound leg extended. Bend the affected knee and hip up to the stomach with the ankle in plantar flexion								

2. Bridging without extension of the affected leg					
3. Extend the affected leg gradually, keeping the ankle dorsiflexed					
4. Dorsiflex the ankle while the hip/knee is extended					

Arm

5. Hand in zero-position. Lift the affected arm up above the head and down again, keeping the elbow extended					
6. The arm by the side. Supinate the forearm					
7. Lift the arm and place the palm of the hand on the opposite shoulder					
8. a) With the arm elevated at 90°, bend the elbow and place palm of the hand on the forehead					
b) Extend elbow and bring arm to the side					

PRONE

1. Up on both elbows					

Figure 2.12 continued

2. a) Bend the affected knee with hip extended

   b) Stop at given points during the movement

3. Hold the affected knee bent at 90°, plantarflex and dorsiflex the ankle

SITTING ON EDGE OF A PLINTH WITHOUT SUPPORT

<u>Arm</u>

1. Protective extension of arms:

   a) Present?

   b) Normal execution?

   c) Normal in time?

2. a) Support on the affected arm						
b) Flex and extend the elbow						

Trunk

1. From supine to sitting on edge of plinth						
2. From standing position to supine on a mat						
3. Turning over from supine to prone towards the sound side						
4. Stand up from supine position on mat						

SITTING ON A CHAIR

1. General impression of sitting position						
2. Feet on floor. Pull the affected foot under the chair						
3. Stand up with the affected foot behind the sound one. No use of hands						

Figure 2.12 continued

4. Sit with arms along the side, hands in zero-position. Lift the affected arm (or both arms together) up above the head and down again, keeping the elbow extended (flexion)				
5. Lift the affected arm extended and outward rotated up above head in abduction and down again				
6. Lift the arm and place the palm of the hand on the opposite shoulder				
7. Elbow at 90°, forearm in zero position (or the arm extended by the side). Flex and extend the fingers				
8. Opposition of thumb against each finger (the same position of the proximal joints as in the previous test)				

GRIP

Testing of strength of grip — independent of the position at the shoulder: Hold a turkish towel in the affected hand. Pt should be able to hold on while the therapist pulls the towel in all directions — out and away from the pt's chest and across the chest

TESTING OF PRECISION

Right hand					
1. Sitting position with forearm supported. Hold a knife/pen. (Lumbrical grip)					
2. Write with pencil					
3. Cut meat					
4. Bring a spoon to the mouth (grip combined with movement of the arm)					

62

Figure 2.12 continued

Left hand

1. Hold a steak with the fork while the (sound) right hand cuts						
2. Bring a fork to the mouth						

Right and left hand

Hold around a large glass and lift it up from table						

STANDING

1. General impression of standing position			
2. Protective extension – forwards:			

a) Present?

b) Normal execution?

c) Normal in time?

3. Balance reactions. Feet parallel. Pt is tipped backwards and is not allowed to take any step:

a) Present?

b) Normal execution?

c) Normal in time?

4. Balance reactions. Pt is tipped to the side. Both sides:

a) Present?

b) Normal execution?

c) Normal in time?

63

Figure 2.12 continued

WITH SUPPORT/WITHOUT SUPPORT

5. Step-position, affected foot in front. Weight transfer on the affected foot. Full transfer by taking a step with the sound leg					
6. Step-position, affected foot behind. Weight transfer on the sound foot (the affected leg rests lightly with the forefoot on the floor, the knee slightly bent and the hip lowered)					
a) Step forward with affected leg. Heel-strike					
7. Stand on affected leg. Make small steps with sound foot forwards and backwards					
8. Stand on sound leg. Make small steps with affected foot forwards and backwards					

WALKING (with cane/elbowcrutch/without support/ with shoe and brace/barefoot)

1. Walk forward with equal steps					
2. Walk backwards					
3. Step over small obstacles — forward/back-ward					
4. Walk up stairs — normal pattern					
5. Walk down stairs — normal pattern (make remark if other pattern)					
6. Running					

GENERAL IMPRESSION:

Date:

Date:

Date:

Figure 2.13 Example of ADL assessment chart.

NAME:
RATING:
0 = Impossible;   * = unaided
1 = Very slow;   † = aided
2 = Mod slow but adequate;
3 = Normal.

Date:
Diagnosis:

	0	1	2	3	REMARKS
1. EVERYDAY ACTIVITIES					
In and out of bed:					
Into bed					
Sit up					
Turn over					
Manage bed clothes					
Out of bed					
Make bed					
2. PERSONAL HYGIENE					
a) Toilet:					
On and off					
Flush					
Manage paper					
Menstruation hygiene					
b) Washing:					
Turning on taps					
Wash hands, face, neck					
Wash hair					
Clean teeth/dentures					

Shave electric/safety
(open, plug in, clean razor)
Brush, comb, part hair
Apply make-up
c) Bathing:
In and out
Down to bottom of bath
Washing/drying extremities
Washing and drying back

3. DRESSING

Patient to dress and undress from
position most used to i.e. bed/chair/
standing. (To be timed)

a) Female:
Bra
Girdle
Pants
Slip
Stockings/tights
Blouse/skirt
Dress
Cardigan
Shoes

Male:
Vest
Shirt
Sweater
Trousers
Socks
Shoes

Figure 2.13 continued

4. FEEDING Cutting up meat Eating with fork/spoon Swallowing Buttering bread Pouring tea Passing plate, tea-cup etc. Holding cup or glass Stirring tea or coffee Lifting mug to mouth	
5. COOKING Beating Breaking eggs Rolling pastry Opening tins Opening screw top jars Washing/peeling veg. Using oven Carrying trays Cutting bread Lifting saucepans Prepare meal	

6. HOUSEWORK

Run house
Washing/drying up
Sweeping/cleaning floor
Dusting/polishing
Washing/wringing/hanging clothes
Laying/lighting fire
Lifting bucket etc.
Sewing/darning/knitting
Lay table/serve meal
Reach shelves

7. UTILITIES

Write/read/speak
Open letters
Manage book/newspaper
Handle money
Use telephone
Wind watch
Thread needle
Use scissors
Operate switches/plugs
Turn doorhandles/knobs
Use keys
Open/close windows

Figure 2.13 continued

8. MOBILITY

a) Wheelchair:
   Transfer forward/side
   Use brakes
   Propel over even/uneven ground
   Propel over ramps/slopes
   Get chair in/out of car

b) On and off chair with arms
   Without arms

c) Pick up objects from floor

d) Walking:
   Indoors — smooth surface
      carpet
      stairs
      lift
   Outdoors — uneven ground/slopes

e) Public transport
      alone
      accompanied

f) Drive car

	TESTS GIVEN (DATE)	SCORE	REMARKS
9. PERCEPTION Constancy — shape — size — colour Scanning Figure ground Position in space Spatial relationships Agnosias — visual — auditory — stereognosis Apraxias — constructional — ideomotor — ideational — dressing Body image — identification — R/L discrimination — neglect			
10. COGNITION Orientation — time — place — person — topographical			

71

Figure 2.13 continued

Memory — short-term
         — recent
         — long-term

Comprehension
Attention span
Reading
Mathematical ability
Money handling
Time telling

FURTHER READING

Assessment

Bobath, B. (1985) *Adult Hemiplegia: Evaluation and Treatment*, William Heinemann Medical Books Ltd., London.

Hemiplegia – assessment and approach, in *Cash's Textbook of Neurology for Physiotherapists*, ch. 10.

Turner, A. (1987) *The Practice of Occupational Therapy*, 2nd edn, Churchill Livingstone, pp.15–38.

Home visit assessment

Turner, A. (1987) *The Practice of Occupational Therapy*, 2nd edn, Churchill Livingstone, pp.143–52.

Assessment tests

Chessington Occupational Therapy Neurological Assessment Battery, available from Nottingham Rehab., Ludlow Hill Rd., West Bridgford, Nottingham, NG2 6HD.

Mahoney, F.I. and Barthel, D.W. (1965) Functional evaluation: Barthel index, *Maryland State Medical Journal*, **14**, 61–5.

Rivermead Assessment Batteries for Activities of Daily Living, Perception, Memory and Unilateral Neglect, available from Rivermead Rehabilitation Unit, Abingdon Rd., Oxford, OX1 4XD.

Turton, A.J. and Frazer, C.M. (1988) A test battery to measure the recovery of voluntary movement control following stroke, *British Journal of Occupational Therapy*, **51**, 1, 11–4.

Wade, D.T. and Collin, C. (1988) The Barthel ADL index: A standard measure of disability?, *International Disability Studies*, **10**, 2, 64–7.

Role of computers in assessment

Feigenson, J.S., McArthy, M.L., Polkow, L., Meikle, R. and Ferguson, W. (1979) Burke Stroke Time-Oriented Profile (BUSTOP): an overview of patient function, *Archives of Physical Medicine Rehabilitation*, **60**, 508–14.

Iverson, J., Sproule, M., Leicht, M., Donald, W.M. and Campbell, D. (1979) Revised Kenny self-care evaluation, *Rehabilitation Publication 722*, Sister Kenny Institute, Minneapolis.

Smith, A.H. (1978) The assessment of patients' prognosis using an interactive computer program, *International Journal of Biomedical Computing*, **9**, 1, 37–44.

Thompson, S.B.N. (1987) A microcomputer-based assessment battery, data file handling and data retrieval system for the forward planning of treatment for adult stroke patients, *Journal of Microcomputer Applications*, **10**, 2, 127–35.

Thompson, S.B.N. and Coleman, M.J. (1987) An interactive microcomputer-based system for the assessment and prognosis of stroke

73

patients. *Paper presented at Special European Conference of the American Society for Cybernetics*, on Design for Development of Social Systems, at the University of St Gallen, Switzerland, 15–19 March 1987 *Journal of Microcomputer Applications*, **12**, no. 1, 33–40.

3

Treatment Approaches

INTRODUCTION

The treatment of stroke patients has become a subject of much controversy in recent years. Developments in our knowledge of stroke have lead to changing attitudes in this area of medicine. The conventional unilateral approach left many patients completely one-sided and one-handed but also relatively if not completely, independent. However, research into neurophysiological techniques has revealed that conventional approaches are not necessarily the best for the patient. But until enough therapists become familiar with these new techniques, OT education will remain biased towards more conventional treatment methods. The result is that treatment regimes remain mixed in many districts.

In any event, gone are the days when every patient was up and walking with whichever aid or gait they could muster; gone are the days when one-handed equipment was issued as a package for stroke patients. The aim for stroke patients was independence at all costs. This was done without fully realizing the disadvantages, such as increased muscle tone, which is detrimental to complete recovery. This often left the patient in pain and discomfort from the tightening spastic limb or trunk muscles.

How much better is the newer neurophysiological approach? Is a mixture of treatment approaches combined with therapist intuition just as effective? Independence should not be sought at the expense of maximum recovery potential, neither should the chosen treatment-approach stifle progress. With stroke patients the therapist should be aiming for independence within the limit of the approach by introducing the patient to the most therapeutic method of carrying out everyday activities at home. Therapists must bear in mind that patients are individuals with personal priorities. The treatment approach must be flexible in order to suit the needs expressed by the patient. In this event, patient motivation will be high and thus the highest level of performance can be expected. The patient's feelings are paramount, as without their co-operation and trust, treatment will fail. The therapist must find the balance between early (probably unilateral) independence and later fully-functional independence. The patient's personality and determination will play a part in deciding which is more important.

For example, a younger patient, strong willed and determined to get up and get going, will do so, sometimes in spite of contrary advice. In these cases, carefully balanced achievement goals can be used to gain co-operation towards the chosen treatment approach. If the reasons for adhering to the chosen approach are explained and the patient understands their importance, this may assist in redressing the balance so that near perfect control of the affected side can be gained.

In the early stages of treatment the approach may be adhered to at the expense of independence. If a patient is referred who is attempting to walk with a one-sided gait and bad posture, they may be confined to a wheelchair temporarily while work is being done to correct this. Self-propelling using one hand or one hand and one foot may additionally be discouraged and the combination of these may frustrate the patient making him/her feel that he/she has taken a backward step in recovery. This is where the time for careful explanation of the reasons for such action is crucial. The patient may also find it difficult to persevere with the learnt techniques outside the therapy sessions. This is where consistency of input from all those involved with the patient will assist. If the patient has difficulty in actually learning the concept this will also limit recovery.

Another example is where a patient may be referred having suffered a stroke many years previously, in which case established routines of one-handed independence may be apparent. In these cases complete revision of techniques will be unnecessary and difficult to attain as the patient is likely to be unwilling or unable to 'unlearn' the old, familiar, techniques. In cases where there are communication problems or poor memory, independence is the primary goal. In addition, if there is severe emotional disturbance (e.g. depression or lability) brought on by the patient's inability to cope with disability, the neurophysiological approach may have to be abandoned.

In both of these situations the honesty of the treatment team will assist in setting realistic, attainable goals of achievement for the patient. This will hopefully maximize motivation for further recovery. There are some key factors to consider in the choice of treatment-approach taken:

1. The patient
   the type and extent of brain damage;
   the age of the spouse or carer;
   comprehension of the patient;
   prognosis;
   any underlying conditions (e.g. heart condition);
   secondary psychological problems such as communication
      difficulties;
   emotional disturbance, or poor motivation;
2. The staff
   consistency of approach and co-operation between the
      disciplines;
   ratio of staff to patients;
   knowledge base;
   experience, background and expertise of staff;
3. The hospital
   organization (e.g. stroke rehabilitation unit or stroke
      patients being treated on a general medical ward);
   the health authority policy (e.g. early discharge or
      maximum level of function prior to discharge);
   facilities (e.g. choice of treatment areas and availability of
      special areas such as a daily living unit for trial period
      prior to discharge);
   staffing levels;
   attitude towards training;
4. Support available
   follow-up at home or outpatient treatment;
   community services available (e.g. district nurse,
      community OT);
   home/family dynamics.

NEUROPHYSIOLOGICAL APPROACHES

Four techniques commonly discussed under the headings of

neurophysiological or neurodevelopmental approach will be discussed in this section: i.e. Bobath, Rood, Brunnström and Proprioceptive Neuromuscular Facilitation (PNF). This section will not advocate use of any particular method but instead present the concepts of each for consideration. It is important to accept that each philosophy is a separate entity and that the designers usually advocate their exclusive use in treating central nervous system disorders. It should also be borne in mind that therapists generally use elements of each of these methods to suit the need of the patient (Collin, 1975).

A survey was carried out by Hurd in 1975 in an attempt to ascertain the use of Bobath and PNF in OT departments. Results showed an increase in interest and awareness of the neurophysiological approaches and indeed this has been the case in ensuing years. Similarly, Hughes (1972) made a comparison of the Bobath and Brunnström methods in an attempt to establish their use in rehabilitation.

Neurophysiological approaches have also been combined under the heading sensory-motor therapy, the principles of which are described in *The Foundation and Practice of Sensory-Motor Therapy* (1986) by Sue Gretton. There are three important factors to consider with neurophysiological approaches:

1. Consistency: a consistent approach between disciplines is essential when applying these techniques. If departments involved in the treatment of stroke patients use different approaches, the patient will not be able to work effectively during treatment. This obviously has training implications on the health service as a whole. Training in techniques such as Bobath or Rood involves attendance on accredited courses (usually by physiotherapists or occupational therapists) followed by internal training sessions for other members of the treatment team: e.g. nursing staff, doctors, therapy assistants, etc. These are costly and time-consuming but nevertheless crucial if these approaches are to be used. Many therapists go ahead and use bilateral activities without the theoretical background knowledge to ensure that they are achieving what is intended or required. This leads to dilution of the correct techniques or bad practice, especially when others copy without learning.

2. Commitment: in contrast to what has already been discussed concerning the balance of approach, commitment to using a

specific approach needs to be established before expecting everyone to implement it – this includes financial commitment of the authority to provide additional staffing. With the unilateral approach many patients were seen by a therapist at the same time. The patients were normally given a task to do and left to get on with it. With neurophysiological approaches, the therapists have to have a one-to-one relationship with the patient whenever possible. The therapist needs to observe and feel what is happening in the muscles, preventing abnormal tone and posture, checking all the time that the patient is doing exactly what is intended, e.g. with weight-bearing to inhibit a spastic upper limb, great care has to be taken that the shoulder joint remains stable and is not subluxed or in spasm. In this way, each person dealing with the patient will understand the necessity of approaching, handling and encouraging the patient to recover in a particular way.

3. Preparatory work plus activity: physiotherapists are trained to move and work patients' limbs in a particular way, towards recovery and control of muscle action following a stroke, especially if using the Bobath approach. On the other hand, occupational therapists are trained to identify deficits in function and to use suitable activities to improve the deficit. The emphasis is therefore on activity. Preparatory work on, for example a limb in spastic tone, is essential before activity can be encouraged. Therapists need to be aware of the necessity for this, but without the addition of a purposeful activity (such as washing, dressing or eating) the treatment is not functional.

With each of the approaches described, a full assessment is carried out prior to implementing the treatment programme. This, as with all patients, is an essential part of the programme to establish where the patient is in recovery and thus how to proceed. It also highlights any problems the patient may have in addition to the hemiplegia/paralysis, e.g. perceptual or cognitive deficits.

The basic principles on which the four treatment approaches are based are:

1. The central nervous system functions appropriately because of the balance between inhibitory and facilitatory influences on the basic motor responses;

2. Specific controlled sensory input can influence motor responses;
3. Abnormal motor responses can be inhibited and more normal motor responses can be learnt by the central nervous system;
4. Proprioceptive and/or exteroceptive stimuli (such as resistance or light brushing, respectively) can be used to influence thresholds for inhibition and facilitation of movement;
5. Reflex mechanisms may be used to facilitate normal movement;
6. Sequences may be based on the recapitulation of ontogenic development.

BOBATH

The Bobath treatment approach as devised by neurologist Dr K. Bobath and physiotherapist Mrs B. Bobath is the most widely adopted. This particular theory and method was devised for children suffering from cerebral palsy (Bobath, 1964; 1967), but the theme was developed and related to patients suffering with strokes and resultant hemiplegia (Bobath, 1959; 1969; 1977; 1985).

Concept

The basic concept behind the treatment approach is that before suffering a stroke, a patient has already developed normally, therefore development of motor control can be gained by:
1. Establishment of reflex postural stability;
2. Regain of control over individual movements by breaking any mass synergistic movement patterns.

Before instigating the treatment regime with the patient, a full assessment will be carried out in the following areas; (a) level of voluntary muscle control, (b) any abnormal responses present, (c) postural tone, and (d) sensation.

Principles of treatment

The two main principles of treatment are: 1. inhibition of unwanted muscle patterns (i.e. the primitive patterns of movements of flexion in the upper limb and extension in the lower limb), and 2. facilitation of the automatic reactions such as righting, equilibrium and protective extension. This is to ensure that the central nervous system is receiving feedback from normal movement. Cortical (voluntary) control is demanded from the patient wherever possible.

Techniques

These principles are achieved by special techniques of handling and positioning (e.g. weight-bearing through an affected upper limb – i.e. a position of extension) in order to:

1. Normalize muscle tone;
2. Elicit the righting and equilibrium responses automatically;
3. Gradually introduce independent voluntary control.

ROOD

Margaret Rood is an occupational therapist and physiotherapist and has concentrated her ideas on the use of sensory stimulation to modify motor patterns in stroke patients (Rood, 1954, 1962; Stockmeyer, 1967; Huss, 1971).

Concept

The concept behind the approach is that motor patterns are developed from fundamental reflex patterns modified through sensory stimuli until the highest control is gained at a conscious cortical level. This being the case, Rood's concept is that if the correct sensory stimulation is applied to sensory receptors, a motor response can be elicited as a reflex, which is then re-established as a normal motor movement pattern.

Principles

The principles of this approach are that:

1. Correct motor output can be gained by correct sensory input;
2. Sensory stimulation is used to promote motor control through the following sequences:
   (a) phasic movement;
   (b) co-contraction patterns around joints for stability;
   (c) heavy work superimposed on the co-contraction leading to weight-bearing;
   (d) skilled co-ordinated movement in a non-weight bearing position with stabilization at proximal joints;
3. The movement is purposeful;
4. Repetition of the sensory-motor experience is necessary for learning the control.

Techniques

1. Controlled sensory stimulation to evoke a response in muscle, e.g. brushing, icing, tapping, quickstretch, joint compression, vibration, etc;
2. Use of a purposeful activity that utilizes the muscle patterns stimulated. The client's attention is thus concentrated on the activity rather than the movements;
3. Use of stimuli to special senses to facilitate or inhibit muscle activity, e.g. visual or auditory stimuli used to promote responses during treatment.

BRUNNSTRÖM

Signe Brunnström is a physical therapist who uses movement therapy in direct contrast to most other methods. She suggests using the abnormal movement patterns in treatment rather than inhibiting them or discouraging their use. In her book *Movement Therapy in Hemiplegia*, she gives a direct account of this particular approach (Brunnström, 1956, 1962, 1966, 1971; Perry, 1967).

Concept

Brunnström's concept is that hemiplegic patients will progress through a defined series of six recovery stages. These follow the development of limb synergies that are primitive patterns of flexion and extension which are normally modified by higher cortical centres of the brain. The six stages are:

1. Flaccidity;
2. Synergies develop such as flexion patterns in the upper limb and extension in the lower limb;
3. Spasticity increases;
4. Some movements deviate from synergy and spasticity is reduced;
5. Independence can be gained from the synergies;
6. Isolated joint movements can occur with co-ordination. Spasticity is not present.

Principles of Treatment

Maximum use should be made of muscles by utilizing the following in treatment rather than inhibiting them:

1. The synergies present in the stroke patients;
2. The exaggerated primitive postural reflexes;
3. The associated reactions (usually considered as abnormal patterns in other treatment approaches).

Techniques

Proprioceptive and exteroceptive stimuli with resistance are applied during the activity to make the patient aware of the sensation of movement, plus specific handling by the therapist during treatment, coupled with verbal commands instructing the patient to perform a particular movement. Examples of this related to the occupational therapy setting would be activities such as sanding, sawing, planing etc. to promote use of limb flexion and extension with resistance.

PROPRIOCEPTIVE NEUROMUSCULAR FACILITATION (PNF)

This treatment approach was initially developed by Herman Kabat and expanded by Margaret Knott (1973) and Dorothy Voss (1959, 1967, 1972). PNF stresses the importance of using resisted movement, manual contacts and voice tones during treatment to reinforce desired movement patterns.

Concept

1. The patients' potential is maximized in response to demands made upon them;
2. Repetition promotes learning (as with Rood);
3. A purposeful activity aiming towards a goal assists in recovery;
4. The stronger muscles stimulate and strengthen the weaker ones. In this approach, the treatment initially calls for use of the strongest and most co-ordinated muscle groups available in the patient.

Principles

1. Functional movement patterns such as postural and righting reflexes are used rather than identifying individual muscle groups, i.e. spiral and diagonal patterns of movement are encouraged;
2. Sensory stimuli are used to assist in obtaining functional movement patterns and muscle strength is used to stimulate proprioception;
3. Maximal resistance (but not over-powering) is used to facilitate patterns.

Techniques

- Icing for inhibition, e.g. cold compresses for reduction of spasticity;
- Positioning, e.g. to support effort or increase demand;
- Manual contacts, e.g. use pressure to place demand on muscles;
- Verbal commands, e.g. strong commands or moderate praise;
- Stretch stimulation, e.g. to elicit antagonistic muscle responses;
- Traction and approximation, e.g. to stimulate joint receptors;
- Maximal resistance, e.g. to elicit maximum effort from the patient;

- Normal timing, e.g. to encourage smooth co-ordinated movements;
- Timing for emphasis, e.g. using stronger muscles to stimulate weaker muscles;
- Repeated contractions, e.g. to strengthen areas needing improvement;
- Hold, relax, active, e.g. a less vigorous version of repeated contractions;
- Slow reversal, e.g. to stimulate the agonistic pattern where this is weaker than the antagonistic pattern;
- Rhythmic stabilization, e.g. where the patient holds against resistance;
- Relaxation.

FURTHER READING

Neurophysiological techniques

Boyd, R.V. (1987) The rehabilitation of stroke illness, *The Practitioner*, **231**, 890–5.

Collin, M.E. (1975) Neurophysiological techniques in the treatment of the adult neurologically impaired patient, *British Journal of Occupational Therapy*, **8**, 166–7.

Hurd, S.N. (1975) Trends in treatment methods and media, including the use of PNF and the Bobath approach. A survey of Occupational Therapy for the hemiplegic patient, *British Journal of Occupational Therapy*, **38**, no. 4, 81–3.

Bobath

Bobath, B. (1977) Treatment of adult hemiplegia, *Physiotherapy*, **63**, 10, 310–3.

Bobath, B. (1985) *Adult Hemiplegia: Evaluation and Treatment*, William Heinemann, London.

Rood

Huss, J. (1971) Sensorimotor treatment approaches, in *Occupational Therapy*, 4th edn, (eds Willard and Spackman), J.B. Lippincott Company, Philadelphia, pp. 380–3.

Rood, M. (1954) Neurophysiological reactions as a basis for physical therapy, *Physical Therapy Review*, **34**, 166–7.

Stockmeyer, S. (1967) An interpretation of the approach of Rood to the treatment of neuromuscular dysfunction, *American Journal of Physical Medicine*, (NUSTEP proceedings), **46**, 1, 900–56.

Brunnström

Brunnström, S. (1956) Associated reactions of the upper extremity in adult patients with hemiplegia. An approach to training, *Physical Therapy Review*, **36**, 225-36.
Brunnström, S. (1970) *Movement Therapy in Hemiplegia*, Harper and Row, New York.

Proprioceptive neuromuscular facilitation (PNF)

Voss, D.E. (1967) PNF, *American Journal of Physical Medicine*, **46**, 1, 838-98.
Voss, D.E. (1972) Proprioceptive neuromuscular facilitation: the PNF method, in *Physical Therapy Services in Developmental Disabilities*, (eds Pearson and Williams), Charles C. Thomas, Springfield, Illinois.

4

Occupational Therapy

Activity is the basis of all treatment in the OT department. The skill of a competent therapist is in making the most appropriate choice of activities suited to the needs and abilities of the patient. Sometimes it may be tempting to disregard the foundations of OT in pursuit of new ideas and approaches, instead of integrating one with the other to establish better practice. Whichever treatment approach is chosen, the basic ideals must remain, i.e. that activity is valuable both in assessment and treatment of stroke patients.

As long as the treatment aims are achieved and the approach is right for the patient, any activity is suitable (depending on the specific function or movement being encouraged). As far as possible, this activity should be functional, purposeful and rewarding to the patient (although in interim stages they may be non-purposeful in order to elicit a specific movement required for a later activity). Also, the activity should not be used as an end-product in itself, especially at the expense of required movements; as with treatment approaches, a balance is always required.

AIMS OF TREATMENT

Aims of treatment should be identified with each patient individually, involving the family and/or carers as appropriate. The treatment aims can then be prioritized according to the importance placed upon them by the patient. Aims of treatment will usually fall into the five areas shown, but not necessarily in the order given (the order will also vary during treatment as the patient reaches new stages of recovery). They should all lead to the overall aim which is to help the patients increase in independence, enabling them to return to as near previous lifestyle as is possible.

Throughout the rehabilitation process, the therapist should be aware of any psychological problems that the patient is suffering. Feelings of frustration, depression or low esteem will hinder the patient's ability to achieve maximum recovery, and lability or personality changes may add to any difficulties that the family may be experiencing. Use of counselling skills (particularly good listening), answering questions honestly, giving advice, explanations and information where required, will all help in gaining the confidence of the patients and their families during treatment. It is important to try and give support where and when necessary, without overloading or smothering them in the process.

The five aims of treatment that are going to be discussed in this chapter are:

1. Improve physical function;
2. Establish independence in activities of daily living (ADL);
3. Alleviate communication problems;
4. Alleviate perceptual problems;
5. Assist in resettlement.

Improve physical function

Inhibiting abnormal patterns of movement to normalize muscle tone and establish correct patterns of functional movement

Positioning Appropriate positioning of the patient within his/her surrounding environment as well as specific positions suitable for treatment activities are extremely important especially in the early stages. In the ward, the bed should be placed so that the locker, food/drink, television, visitors and objects of interest are on the patient's affected side. This will encourage awareness of that side which is an essential step towards recovery.

Reflex inhibiting patterns The following patterns of movement should be encouraged as far as possible before attempting treatment activities. This is where the preparatory work can make a difference to the achievements of a treatment session.

Where there is abnormal flexor muscle tone in the trunk and arm, the following patterns are required:

- Extension of neck and spine;
- External rotation of arm at shoulder and abduction;
- Extension of elbow;
- Extension of wrist with supination;
- Abduction of thumb.

Where there is abnormal extensor and flexor muscle tone in leg:

- Abduction with external rotation;
- Extension of hip;
- Slight flexion at knee;
- Dorsiflexion of toes and ankle;
- Abduction of big toe.

Where there is abnormal muscle tone of the trunk:

- Rotation of shoulder girdle against pelvis;
- Rotation of pelvic girdle against shoulder.

When assisting the patient to sit up from lying, care should be taken not to damage the patient's shoulder or the carer's back. If the correct procedure is carried out this will not happen. The patient is rolled onto the affected side. The therapist then puts one hand under the affected side at the shoulder and the other hand over the patient's legs. The therapist then swings the patient's legs over the side of the bed, at the same time supporting the shoulder as the patient swings into the sitting position. During this phase elongation of the trunk occurs and if a pause is needed to re-arrange clothing, the patient can be propped on the affected elbow and take weight through the upper limb.

When sitting in a chair for activities of daily living or specific treatment activities, the patient should sit well back in the chair with hips, knees and ankles at 90°. The head and trunk should be in line, with body weight evenly distributed on both buttocks. The affected upper limb should be protracted at the shoulder and supported forward on a table or pillow, including the hand and wrist (the patient should be discouraged from 'cradling' his/her arm as this will encourage spasticity).

Treatment activities to assist in improving physical function It is extremely important for the therapist to explain the relevance of each activity both before and during the treatment session. These

89

should be carried out after suitable preparatory work has been done on head and trunk control or weight-bearing position. Activities may be carried out with the patient sitting or standing at a table, or using the floor as an activity area. The aims of these activities are:

* To encourage reaching forwards, down, up and to the side;
* To improve sitting or standing balance;
* To improve general co-ordination.

Examples of activities (these activities can be done bilaterally or by weight-bearing through the affected upper limb progressing onto unilateral work with the affected upper limb):

* Scoring floor target to throw items from varying distances;
* Draughts or noughts-and-crosses, with a variety of positions to work at and different sized pieces;
* Large bilateral shove-ha'penny;
* Large number game board with bilateral handle grips on pieces (Eggers, 1983);
* Sanding, polishing or cleaning work surfaces after cookery, art, craft or heavy workshop activities;
* Popomatic dice machine for use with any table game involving dice throwing;
* Hoopla or skittles, especially to promote standing balance whilst reaching down and swinging forward at the same time. Skittles can be played using a large ball to begin with, and the players either sitting or standing;
* Croquet arches using a long-handled mallet, bilaterally at first, to push the balls through a row of wooden arches. This can be transferred to outdoor croquet to encourage walking and balancing on uneven surfaces.

Examples of activities used to help the return of upper limb function are:

* Draughts, span games, foot draughts (with hand slid through straps), which can be used to promote shoulder control, initially played on the floor, progressing to elevating the activities;
* Draughts, solitaire, Connect-4, marbles, for grip and release, and pronation and supination;

- Bagatelle, popomatic dice, shove-ha'penny, for finger extension;
- Jigsaws, jacks, three-dimensional Connect-4, cards, for improving fine finger dexterity. Jigsaws, in particular, are also useful for promoting discussion and improving perception;
- Typing or computer keyboard skills for improving fine finger dexterity, and hand-eye co-ordination.

The following are examples of activities used to help the return of lower limb function:

- Croquet arches, kicking the ball through the arches, helps to prepare for the swing phase of the walking gait;
- Foot draughts, foot noughts-and-crosses (initially sitting, then standing);
- Heavy workshop activities (see next aim).

The following are examples of activities used to improve general mobility, balance and upper limb control and co-ordination:

- Heavy workshop activities such as bench work, planing, sawing, sanding, varnishing, painting and general use of tools. Care should be taken not to add resistance to activities (unless the Brunnström approach is being used). It is also vital to establish individuals on a one-to-one basis with separate specific instructions concerning work position and use of tools and materials. Motivation will be improved if a choice of project is offered;
- Printing: throughout the processes of composing, printing-off and laying-out, a variety of positions can be used to suit each patient's needs, e.g. composing can be done seated or standing, weight-bearing or unilaterally;
- Office skills (e.g. duplicating, collating, guillotining, stapling, etc.); as with printing, these can be done either weight-bearing or bilaterally progressing to unilaterally.

Improving sensation, proprioception and stereognosis

These can all be improved during practise in activities of daily living and through remedial activities. Two examples are:

1. Dressing and washing
   Sensation: encourage the patient to remark on textures of different types of clothing, and check temperature sensation when running water for a wash;
   Stereognosis: ask the patient to identify objects with his/her eyes closed; for example, soap, flannel, toothbrush, etc;
   Proprioception: watch the patient's responses to commands for particular actions during activities such as fastenings behind the back, or tucking in shirt/blouse.
2. Remedial activities
   Sensation: activities such as gardening (where the patient mixes sand and soil to fill pots and seed trays), cooking (particularly bread-making or any other recipes requiring hand manipulation of ingredients), crafts (working with beads, wool, leather, collage materials, etc.) or specific remedial games such as matching textures dominoes improves sensitivity of the hands and fingers plus general co-ordination and dexterity;
   Stereognosis: identifying objects by feel behind a screen or in bags (this can be done as a game, keeping score of the number of correct identifications for future reference);
   Proprioception: exercises to music such as 'Simon Says ...', where the patient responds to requests made by the therapist. The patient should be encouraged to appreciate when the correct position is made so that he/she will know which position to relate to which request.

Establishing methods of transfer

1. Assisted transfers (sitting to sitting): e.g. chair, toilet, stool, edge of bed, car. During these transfers the therapist should always remember to bend at the knees and not at the back to avoid straining. Transferring in the way described, emphasizes the patient's affected side, encouraging him/her to take notice of it and take weight through it.

- The patient should move as far forward in the chair as possible by hip hitching, so that his/her feet are flat on the floor;
- The patient should interlock the fingers and extend the arms out in front – the patient's feet should be slightly apart with the affected foot slightly behind. This is so that when he/she

stands, the initial weight will be taken through the affected leg;

- The therapist stands in front of the patient. His/her arms are placed under the patient's axilla on the unaffected side and round the affected arm, with hands flat over the scapulae. The therapist's legs are either side of the patient's affected leg, blocking the knee and foot;
- The patient's trunk is brought forward and he/she is brought to standing so that the body weight is taken equally through both legs. No attempt is made to lift the body weight at all and the therapist's body counterbalances that of the patient;
- To move round to the surface being transferred to, the therapist slides the patient's affected foot round with his/her own, the patient stepping round with the unaffected foot. When able the patient can step round with both feet;
- To return to sitting the patient should be back far enough to feel the chair seat on the back of his/her legs. The patient should then lean forward, bending at the waist and hip, with his/her bottom sticking out, and slowly lowering him/herself down into the chair.

2. Independent transfers

(a) Sitting-to-standing

- When standing from sitting; weight should be kept forward, the head vertically over, or a little in front of the feet and the weight equally distributed over both feet, with the affected leg slightly behind;
- The hands are clasped together, fingers interlaced and both arms are pulled forward in front of the knees to assist balance; extension, causing a thrust-back of the patient's weight, should be discouraged and the patient should try to maintain the weight in the midline;
- Once the body weight is raised from the seat, the bottom should be tucked in and the patient straightened up keeping weight central;
- When standing, the patient should pivot, as far as necessary, towards the other seat;
- The patient should feel for the seat against the back of his/her legs and look behind so that he/she is sure where he/she is going. The patient should not reach for the arm of the chair, but;

- Reversing the sitting-to-standing procedure with hips and knees flexed, he/she should keep the head and arms well forward, lower bottom onto the seat keeping the weight over both feet (affected foot slightly behind to encourage weight taken through that leg).

When perfected, this technique enables a sitting-to-sitting transfer without the assistance of any aids, or gadgets for maintaining balance. It can therefore be used safely for transferring on and off car seats, toilets, stools, etc.

(b) Bed transfers – into bed

- The bedcovers should be pulled back and the patient should be in a sitting position on the side of the bed, with the affected side towards the pillow;
- The patient leans to the affected side, taking weight through the affected upper limb; either with outstretched arm which is then lowered to take weight on the elbow and forearm, or, if there is not enough control of the elbow, straight to elbow and forearm;
- While going down onto the affected side the patient swings the legs up onto the bed. If the affected leg cannot reach the bed independently then it can be assisted by the unaffected arm while stabilizing the body on the bed with the unaffected leg;
- When the patient is lying on the affected side; the leg underneath should be positioned in extension at the hip before the covers are pulled up. The arm which is underneath should be positioned with the shoulder protracted, the arm and forearm either outstretched or bent up onto the pillow. The unaffected leg is flexed at the hip and knee to maintain position with comfort;
- If the patient is lying on the unaffected side, the top leg is positioned in front flexed at the knee and hip, resting on a pillow to avoid falling into medial rotation at the hip and inversion at the ankle. Again, the affected shoulder should be pulled forward into protraction and rested on the pillow.

(c) Bed transfers – out of bed

- From lying on the affected side, the lower limbs should be

flexed at the hip and knee, bringing them to the end of the
bed;

- The trunk is pushed up into the side sitting position, with
  weight on the affected elbow. The unaffected hand should be
  placed in front of the body near the affected elbow;
- As the patient raises his/her trunk to the sitting position, the
  legs should be swung off the bed onto the floor;
- Sitting balance should be established with the feet correctly
  positioned before the patient attempts to stand up.

(d) Other bed transfers

If the bed has to be approached from the other side then:

(i) Getting in:

The patient should start in a sitting position, angled a little down
the bed, with the back towards the pillows;

The patient lowers him/herself onto the affected side with the
upper trunk angled across the bed and towards the pillows;

The legs are swung up, flexed at the hip to get them onto the
bed;

The body is then straightened to get the head to the top of the
bed.

(ii) Getting out:

The patient should lie on the affected side, bent at the hips so
that his/her body is angled across the bed, with the bottom near
the edge of the bed;

The patient should push into a sitting position and swing the
legs to the side and back off the bed until he/she is sitting angled
on the edge of the bed;

Sitting balance should be established, with the feet correctly
positioned before the patient stands up.

3. Bath transfers

(a) Using a board and seat

- The patient should position a chair alongside the bath and
  transfer to sitting on the bath board as for sitting-to-sitting
  transfer as described above;
- The patient lifts each leg into the bath separately, maintaining

sitting balance on the bath board;

- Keeping both knees flexed and feet securely on the bath mat (taking weight through both feet) the patient should lower him/herself onto the bath seat by holding the side of the bath with the unaffected hand keeping the affected upper limb inhibited;
- If the patient wishes to go right into the bath, he/she follows the same procedure again;
- If the patient wishes, the bath board and seat may now be removed while the patient washes, and returned again for getting out;
- To get out of the bath, the patient does the reverse movements making sure that both knees are flexed and feet are flat on the bath mat. If necessary, a carer can assist by holding the affected knee flexed to prevent the leg from shooting forward into extension as the patient moves up onto the seat or board.

(b) Getting in (without board or seat)

This method can be attempted as soon as the patient can get him/herself off the floor, through kneeling, using a chair or stool for assistance. A non-slip rubber bath mat is usually used for safety.

It is preferable to start from a position facing the tap end of the bath, irrespective of the side affected. However, some patients prefer to lead with the unaffected side and therefore would start with back to the taps and turn round in the bath before sitting down:

- Standing beside the bath, the patient leans forward and places both hands on the rim of the bath. The unaffected hand maintains the position of the affected hand, and grasp of both;
- Taking full weight on the leg furthest from the bath, the patient lifts the other leg into the bath and positions it firmly in the middle of the bath width, to take the body weight;
- The patient transfers his/her body weight to the leg in the bath and lifts the second leg in;
- The patient should ensure that balance is held firmly on both feet, before letting go with the hands to stand up – keeping weight central, the patient bends the knees and hips and lowers to a sitting position in the bath. The hands should be

grasped hands together and the patient should lean forward so that arms and head are vertically in front of the feet, until ready to sit back.

(c) Getting out (without board or seat)

- The patient sits up in the bath and bends knees up towards the chest;
- The unaffected hand is placed behind the patient in the bath to take weight;
- The patient leans trunk towards unaffected side so that the shoulders and hips face sideways within the bath, and knees are tucked up and angled towards the back of the bath;
- The affected knee is pulled through so that it faces towards the back corner, with help from the unaffected arm if necessary. The affected foot should be in front of the unaffected foot;
- The patient edges further round so that the shoulders are facing towards the back of the bath, the knees edged round as far as possible;
- The patient then leans the head and shoulders forward, turns right round to the back of the bath, pulls up onto the knees with both hands on the floor of the bath to stabilize him/herself;
- The hands are brought up to the back rim of the bath and the patient kneels up straight;
- One leg is brought up into half-kneeling and the patient stands, keeping weight forward;
- The hands are transferred to the side rim of the bath (as for getting in);
- The weight is taken through the leg nearest to the wall side of the bath and the other is taken out;
- The weight is transferred onto the leg outside the bath and the second leg is lifted out before the patient stands up.

Establishing method of mobility

Guidelines for minimal requirements for independent walking and wheelchair management are given in Tables 4.1 and 4.2 from Savinelli *et al.* (1978). They give an indication of the level of control and co-ordination required in all the physical assessment areas before independent function can be expected.

Table 4.1
Minimal requirements for independent walking
(adapted from Savanelli *et al.*, 1978)

Cognitive ability to initiate and perform safely
Energy capacity to meet the specific physiological demands
created during walking
Motor control adequate to meet postural demands

Muscle strength and control criteria

Neck — fair; Trunk — poor;
Unaffected upper limb — good if used for support;
Unaffected lower limb — good to normal;
Affected lower limb;
    Stance:
      Hip   — adequate extension to prevent uncontrolled
               forward lean of the trunk;
              — adequate lateral stability to prevent loss of single
               limb balance or use of a walking stick to substitute
               for lateral/forward hip instability;
      Knee — adequate extension to support body weight on a
               flexed knee or adequate control to extend the knee
               prior to full weight acceptance;
      Ankle — adequate plantar flexion or substitution to prevent
               forward collapse of tibia.
    Swing: Adequate limb flexion or substitution to clear toe;

Range of movement

    Stance:
            — centre of trunk mass aligned over feet or adequate
               compensatory posture;
            — no greater than 15° hip flexion contracture unless
               hip extension strength is adequate to compensate;
            — full knee extension unless adequate hip and knee
               extension and/or plantar flexion strength to
               compensate;
            — plantigrade foot; may be achieved by use of foot
               drop splint.

Spasticity

       — extensor tone does not prevent flexion or compensatory
         motion during swing, cause loss of balance or create
         ankle/foot instability during stance;
       — flexion tone does not prevent placement of foot on floor;
       — adduction tone does not cause limb placement beyond
         midline.

Balance

       — 2 limb momentary standing balance without hand support
         or single limb standing balance with hand support.

Sensation

    — Proprioception deficit compensated for by vision or use of splint.

Perceptual integration

    — awareness of body parts;
    — awareness of body position in space;
    — motor planning skills for gross total body activity;
    — visual integration for safe function in the environment.

Table 4.2
Minimal requirements for independent wheelchair management (adapted from Savanelli *et al.*, 1978)

Cognitive ability to initiate and perform safely
Energy capacity to meet the specific physiological demands for propulsion and standing
Motor control adequate to meet postural demands.
Muscle strength and control criteria
Neck — fair; Trunk — poor
Unaffected upper limb — good
Unaffected lower limb — good to normal
                  fair to good for non-postural muscles.

Range of motion

Unaffected upper limb and lower limb — within normal limits;
Affected upper limb — not significant;
Affected lower limb — 110° hip flexion.

Spasticity

    — extensor tone does not prevent trunk, hip and knee flexion to get trunk aligned over feet to arise from sitting;
    — adduction tone does not cause limb placement beyond midline.

Balance

    — independent functional sitting balance;
    — single or 2 limb momentary standing balance without hand support

Sensation

    — proprioception deficit compensated for by vision or use of splint.

Perceptual integration

    — awareness of body parts;
    — awareness of body position in space;
    — motor planning skills for gross total body activity;
    — visual integration for safe function in the environment.

Walking aids The use of walking aids with stroke patients is decreasing as the emphasis remains on regaining full muscle control as early as possible. However, walking aids may be indicated in certain cases:

- For early bilateral walking training (e.g. forearm bilateral walker with wheels or bilateral Zimmer walking frame);
- Where progress in walking is affected by lack of confidence, poor balance or perceptual disorders (e.g. walking stick, quadpod, tripod);
- Where prolonged weakness indicates support is required on a long-term basis (e.g. walking stick, quadpod, tripod).

Wheelchairs As mentioned in Chapter 3 (page 76), it may not be desirable for a patient to self-propel in a wheelchair if increased tone is apparent. However, there are two incidences where use of a wheelchair may be recommended:

- As a mobility aid for therapists and nurses on the ward;
- To provide a correctly-adapted treatment base which encourages good posture and positions for rest or therapy.

The patient should be assessed for a wheelchair that can be used until a decision is made regarding his/her potential for walking. However, if progress is slow and the affected side remains flaccid, one-handed wheelchair mobility may be required as a longer term measure.

Where self-propelling is not desirable due to increased tone, some examples of suitable wheelchair models are as follows:

- A 9L (with all four small wheels) to discourage the patient completely, or
- An 8BL/8L if the patient is able to maintain his/her own decreased tone, but independent mobility is desirable.

Where self-propelling is desirable due to a prolonged flaccid stage or recovery of balance/posture control is limited:

- A double rim one-handed Carter's wheelchair;
- An ARNAS wheelchair;
- A foot steering wheelchair.

Assessment in all cases should consider the patient's need for a chair and not fitting an available chair to the patient. The following variations on wheelchair features may be considered:

- Seat: size, height, and width;
- Cushioning: (Borello-France *et al.*, 1988);
- Backrest: angle and folding mechanism;
- Footrest: length, use of heel straps, whether removable ones are required;
- Wheels: large rear wheels for self-propelling, front castors for manoeuvrability;
- Armrests: special fitments to support a flaccid upper limb, for example, Steed cushion (Steed, 1986), or sling (Davies and Knapp, 1986);
- Tray: this can also be used to support affected arm in position of inhibition. Overall size, weight, folding mechanism (if to be transported in a car);
- Home situation: also needs to be checked as access through doors and some rooms may be required at home.

Prevent deformity

The best way to prevent deformity is through positioning as previously discussed on page 88; (Inhibiting abnormal patterns of movement). In some cases splinting may be indicated to maintain the correct position and prevent permanent deformity such as contractures.

Anti-spastic splints These should not be needed if correct positioning is encouraged from the very beginning of rehabilitation. However, they may be indicated in the following cases:

- If marked increased tone is present;
- If safety is a problem with a very flaccid arm which is susceptible to being caught in the spokes of a wheelchair or trapped down the side of a chair.

Examples are inflatable arm splints or forearm gutters attached to the arm rest (with or without cone-shaped hand grip).

Foot drop splints These may be indicated at the compromise stage when progress in walking is affected by lack of return of effective dorsiflexion in the ankle. Again, as a protective measure, it may be used to prevent inversion of the foot where weight will be taken on the lateral border of the foot. This puts extra stress on the lateral ligaments of the ankle joint and leads to unsteady gait and the possibility of falls.

Home management

Domestic ADL The aim in domestic work as with personal independence is to involve the affected side in the activity as much as possible without making the task impractically difficult or unsafe. A good standing posture should always be encouraged; the body weight being taken evenly through both lower limbs and the patient facing square on to the activity, not side on with the affected side a little back from the activity (which the patient may feel is more comfortable).

When sitting to do domestic work, if the upper limb is not assisting in active function, it should be held in a position of inhibition. Whenever possible it should be involved in active function, either stabilizing or supporting the work done with the unaffected hand. For example, when cooking, a mixing bowl can be placed on a non-slip mat for safety but it can still be stabilized a little by the affected hand. Activities that involve gross movement should be undertaken bilaterally, e.g. folding laundry. In most domestic activities, the affected upper limb can be involved in some way and the patient should be encouraged to do this whenever possible. However, where heat is involved, e.g. ironing and cooking, the patient should be alert to the dangers of impaired sensation or proprioception.

Hints for one-handed kitchen work Useful ideas for one handed kitchen work can be found in *Kitchen Sense for Disabled and Elderly People* available from the Disabled Living Foundation, 346 Kensington High Street, London W14. Some useful suggestions are:

- to stabilize bowls, plates, etc., they can be placed on a dycem mat or held between the knees if the patient is seated. The affected side should be used as a stabilizer wherever possible;
- spike-boards can be used to secure vegetables and fruit when peeling, or the food cooked and skins removed later (e.g. jacket potatoes or sieved stewed apple);
- a full saucepan or kettle on the back of the stove will steady a

saucepan that is being stirred if it is pushed back against the weight at the back of the stove;

- a rubber-sucker soap pad in the washing up bowl will stabilize saucepans while scrubbing them;
- washing up can be saved by soaking pans immediately after use so that food does not harden in the pan. Similarly, non-stick pans or well-greased baking tins will make cleaning easier;
- items can be left to drain rather than drying up;
- hand-mixing can be tiring one-handed. It can help to warm ingredients first and mix-in in small quantities. If available, an electric mixer can be of use;
- labour saving techniques should be used in the kitchen, e.g. slide heavy objects along work surfaces instead of lifting, get all ingredients out before starting work, use convenience foods such as dried onions, frozen pastry, sliced bread, instant potato;
- perching stools can be used rather than standing all the time, if the patient can balance safely whilst using one;
- when making small cakes in bun tins, the spoon can be dipped in hot water first so that the mixture drops off easily, or an ice-cream scoop can be used;
- butter should be kept out of the fridge for a short while before use, or margarine can be used so that spreading bread is easier. A bread-spreading board may prove useful;
- to help when draining vegetables, cook them in a chip basket in the saucepan or use a vegetable draining basket;
- eggs can be cracked on the side of the bowl and opened by pulling them apart using the thumb and fourth and fifth fingers;
- eggs can be separated by cracking them into a saucer, covering the yolk with an egg cup and holding it in place while pouring the white off;
- a trolley or apron with large pockets will save the necessity of carrying things about;
- milk bottle carriers are also useful for carrying other bottles and glasses;
- to open jars, the jars can be held between the knees or wedged in a drawer, or held between the body and the work surface. Alternatively, electric tin openers (one-handed or wall-mounted) or use of a belli-clamp or twister/opener may be advised;

- foods which are used regularly should be transferred into easily opened containers.

Housework, laundry and shopping It is necessary to identify those activities which are essential for the patient to achieve in order to maintain him/herself at home. Most activities involved can be done bilaterally if indicated, or unilaterally with the unaffected side if tone is not increased (e.g. vacuuming, loading washing machine, etc.). Some activities can be used to reinforce treatment already being carried out. This can be done if the correct positions and techniques are taught and practised in the occupational therapy department before returning home (e.g. washing up, hand washing, dusting and polishing, where both hands are used in rhythmical movements with shoulders forward and elbows and wrists extended – i.e. in a position of inhibition). The patient should be given the opportunity to practise any activity enough to master it to his/her satisfaction before attempting it at home. Any particular problems may be overcome in time by the patient him/herself finding a suitable solution. However, in cases where recovery is prolonged, or balance or perceptual problems make domestic activities dangerous, help should be arranged, either privately or through the Social Services Department.

A good pre-discharge indicator is assessment of a patient's ability to shop for, prepare and cook a meal for themselves. At first this activity may be broken down into stages and practised until the patient can manage the whole task themselves. An ideal situation is where a patient can spend some time in a unit such as an independent-living bungalow for a few days prior to going home. Any problems in any of the areas of ADL can then be highlighted and overcome before a final discharge date is set.

Establish independence in activities of daily living (ADL)

Personal activities of daily living

Undressing (i.e. nightwear) It is helpful to untie pyjama trousers before transferring from the bed to a chair, or lifting the nightdress so that it is not sat upon. To remove the pyjama jacket, it should be pushed backwards off the affected shoulder, then the unaffected one. The sleeve should be shaken-off the unaffected arm and then pulled off the affected arm. To remove a nightdress the patient should reach to the back of the neck with the unaffected hand and pull the garment over the head. Again, the unaffected arm should be removed first followed by the affected one.

Dressing While using established one-handed dressing techniques, the patient should be encouraged to maintain a symmetrical sitting or standing posture, to be aware of the affected side and its position and to use whatever function there is in the affected side to its maximum.

Dressing from a sitting position; it is preferable to sit on the edge of the bed rather than a chair, especially one with arms, as there is then more room for arm movement and the affected upper limb is not encouraged into a flexed pattern. Similarly, sitting balance must be established and maintained, rather than leaning against the back or side of a chair. Clothes placed on the affected side encourage awareness of that side as well as exercising compensation for visual complication, i.e. hemianopia. If the clothes are arranged in sequence or marked in a particular way, this can help the patient put them on in the correct order. Also, some patients may find it easier to manage lower garments whilst lying on the bed. In this position, for example, bridging or rolling from side-to-side can make pulling up trousers much easier. The choice of clothes may also make dressing easier. Initially, familiar everyday clothes should be brought in for the patient rather than best wear. Track suits and leisure wear tend to prove popular and easy to manage.

As much active movement as possible should be encouraged. If there is enough shoulder movement to aim the affected hand at the armhole inside a jumper without assistance from the other, then the unaffected arm can be straightening the clothing, making the process quicker and easier. Similarly with feet, the patient must be encouraged to raise the affected leg actively rather than lifting it over.

If the patient has been taught to stand from sitting without pushing or pulling on any aid, then the maintenance of balance in a flexed position, pulling up clothes as he straightens produces no new problem; but with a little practice can be managed using the same techniques as taught for standing from sitting.

The patient may take an extraordinarily long time to dress, or it may be very tiring. If there is help available at home, this will preserve the patient's energy for the rest of the day. It is not necessary to make the patient totally independent in washing and dressing skills if it means that half the day is taken up and the patient is not able to enjoy the rest of the day. It is also important to ensure warmth and privacy for patients whilst they are dressing. The use of aids to daily living may help to keep the time taken to a minimum, for example, pick-up stick, long handled shoe-horn, 'no-bows' laces, elastic laces, button hook, or adaptations to clothing.

Underpants/trousers on and off Fabric choice and type of fastening is an important consideration. For women, shiny satin fabrics with large openings (e.g. french knickers) are often easier to manage than traditional cotton pants. Pants or trouser fastenings may be adapted with velcro to open at the side or front. Pants can be attached to the inside of the waistband of skirts or trousers which allows them to be pulled up together with the outer garment when standing. The following method can be used:

- inhibition of the arm and trunk should be maintained whilst dressing the lower half;
- the affected leg can be crossed-over the unaffected leg by interlocking the fingers and lifting just below the affected knee;
- the trousers can now be pulled onto the affected leg up to the knee;
- the unaffected leg can now be put in and both sides pulled up as far as possible;
- the patient should now wriggle from side to side pulling up the trousers, standing up to pull into final position;
- fastenings can be done sitting or standing;
- to remove, the above procedure should be reversed.

Vest/jumper on and off The patient should be advised to have a larger size than usual with large armholes and loose-fitting waist bands. The following method can be used:

- keeping the affected shoulder well forward, the affected arm should be inhibited by the therapist or the affected hand kept on the affected knee;
- the affected arm's sleeve should be hung down between the patient's legs to put the affected arm in and whilst pulling it up above the elbow;
- the unaffected arm can then be placed into the other sleeve

and the garment pulled over the head and straightened into a comfortable position;

* to remove, the garment should be gathered up from the back and pulled over the head. The unaffected arm should be removed first and placed into an inhibitory position, whilst the affected arm is removed from the garment.

Brassière This is usually the most difficult article of clothing to manage. If the patient prefers to wear a bra, then front-opening bras can be easier to manage. Alternatively, the bra can be done up first and put on in the same way as a jumper. An extra length of elastic on the fastening may assist if this method is preferred.

Blouse/shirt/cardigan Loose-fitting items are easier to manage, and slippery fabrics may also help. Cuff fastening on the unaffected side sleeve can be adapted with elastic or long shanks on the buttons. The following method can be used:

* the affected arm should be put into the sleeve first and pulled up over the elbow;
* the garment is passed around the back and the unaffected arm placed into the other sleeve;
* the garment can then be pulled up over the shoulders and straightened before doing the buttons;
* to remove, the buttons should be undone, the unaffected arm taken out, the garment pulled back round towards the affected side and pulled off the affected arm. It is important to keep the affected arm inhibited.

Dress A pinafore dress over a jumper or blouse with front fastening may be recommended. Again, loose fitting slippery fabrics tend to be easier to manage. Ordinary dress fastenings may be adapted to a side velcro-opening or a long cord attached to the zip at the back of the dress. If the dress is loose enough it may be easier to put on over the head as with a jumper.

Skirt This can be put on over the head as for a jumper after putting on the blouse. In this way the blouse will automatically be tucked-in as the skirt is pulled into place.

Tights/stockings The affected foot should be put in first and the tights' legs worked up to the knees. Both sides can then be gradually worked up until in position. 'Hold-up' stockings may be easier, or with longer length dresses or skirts, socks in tight material may be preferred.

Shoes It is especially important for patients who are ambulant to have well fitting and supportive shoes. Slip-on shoes remove the necessity for laces, but if the shoes are lace-up, elastic laces or 'no-bows' laces may be fitted. Buckled shoes can be adapted with velcro. A long handled shoe-horn may assist with getting shoes on and off.

Washing The patient should be sitting in a chair at the sink or with a basin. The patient should retain the correct sitting position whilst washing and have the wash kit on the affected side to encourage him/her to look to that side. The patient should be able to wash the top half independently, the only difficulty being to wash under the affected arm. To do this he/she should lean forwards so that the arm hangs down straight at the side of the affected leg keeping the shoulder protracted. To wash the lower half, the patient should wash as much as possible whilst sitting maintaining inhibition of the affected arm. When the patient needs to stand, the carer should help him/her to maintain standing correctly so that he/she can wash between the legs him/herself. This will help maintain dignity. Alternatively, if the patient is sat on a towel to begin with, he/she may be able to slide forward slightly to wash this area.

Toileting Transfer should be undertaken as for a chair. If there is insufficient room to transfer correctly, the patient should transfer onto a glideabout commode in a larger room and then be wheeled over the toilet and the brakes applied. If a commode is not required, a raised toilet seat may be used if the toilet seat is too low for the patient to stand up from. In addition, a grab rail fitted to the wall on the unaffected side may provide extra support and ensure safety.

As regards cleaning; spring loaded, or single sheet paper dispensers or dispensers with serrated edge paper are most suitable. If necessary, a long-handled paper holder or pick-up stick (especially reserved for the purpose) may be used to hold the paper in a suitable position for cleaning.

To dress again when finished the patient should draw clothing up to the knees before standing up to make completion of dressing easier. The therapist can help ensuring that clothes fastenings can be managed independently. For ladies, dresses should be tucked into bras to keep the dress out of the way.

Finally, to wash and dry hands, automatic water spray taps and hot airdryers can be very useful, or soap can be fixed to suction pads and roller towels used for drying.

Bathing Bath transfers have already been discussed on page 95 (Aim (i) (a)). Other areas to consider are:

- putting in the plug and turning on taps – the patient should sit on a chair near to the tap-end of the bath before reaching in. The plug may be attached to a chain or bar so that the patient doesn't have to reach right down to the bottom of the bath;
- washing hair: use shower attachment hose if available and push-top shampoo dispensers;
- drying hair: it is advisable to keep a style that is easy to manage, unless someone is available to set or blow dry the hair;
- washing: use a long-handled sponge or brush with liquid soap or soap mitts. Soap could also be kept on a magnetic or suction holder, or left as soap on a rope;
- drying: to avoid getting cold while drying, the bathroom should be warm. To help drying, the patient could use a towelling bath robe or use roller towels.

Feeding Until there is enough strength and control in the affected upper limb to manipulate an eating utensil or even to help stabilize the plate, the limb should be placed outstretched on the table with the shoulder protracted, elbow extended as far as is comfortably possible, forearm pronated and hand flat on the table with fingers extended (i.e. in a position of inhibition). As soon as possible the affected arm should be actively brought into feeding with padded handles to assist weak-grip if only used to stabilize the food whilst cutting with the unaffected hand. Other useful aids to eating are combined spoon/forks, non-slip mats and plate guards. Heated plates can be used to keep food warm. The patient can then have small portions and hot second-helpings if required (Morgan, 1986).

Alleviate communication problems

The most common communication problems are described in Chapter 2, page 28 (Assessment). The following ideas should be practised when the therapist is communicating with stroke patients:

- the stroke patient must be treated as an adult even though he/she may have no speech or communication method;
- before speaking to the patient, his/her full attention should be gained;
- try to remember that the patient is not necessarily deaf. Shouting does not improve patient's comprehension. In most cases it will make the patient more confused. The therapist should be aware of possible loss of comprehension;
- some patients will show a good degree of social cover (i.e. they may appear to be using appropriate conversation without really responding accurately to the therapist) and it is important to be aware of this when it is occurring;
- the therapist should be aware of possible yes/no confusion. Many patients will nod their head while saying no, while some will produce both yes and no in response to a question. Gestural responses are usually more reliable;
- sentences and requests should be kept short and simple. Complex structures or abstract terms should be avoided;
- it may be necessary to repeat the statement two or three times in order for the patient to comprehend what the therapist is trying to say;
- the patient requires plenty of time to decode incoming information, especially if comprehension is limited;
- the therapist should use appropriate gestures to reinforce what is being said to the patient;
- initially it may help if the therapist uses closed questions, i.e. questions requiring only yes/no answers;
- if all else fails, write down the request or statement, or perhaps just the key words. Every opportunity for stimulation should be attempted, e.g. visual, auditory, gestural and tactile.

The following ideas may help the patient express him/herself:

- minimize jargon (e.g. nonsensical syllables or sentences);
- do not reinforce recurrent utterances;

- encourage social speech such as exchanging greetings;
- encourage automatic speech such as counting, days of the week, etc.;
- encourage the patient to repeat simple words that are appropriate to his/her surroundings or needs;
- the therapist should use simple verbal cues to elicit single words from the patient;
- the use of phrases or short sentences should be encouraged where appropriate. These sentences can be repeated back to the patient using the correct grammatical structure without making it obvious that he/she is being corrected.

Alleviate perceptual problems

Most occupational therapists use what is known as the functional approach to the treatment of perceptual deficits (Siev and Freishstat, 1970). This approach recommends the repetition of particular tasks, usually activities of daily living, which will make the patient more independent in meeting his/her basic needs. The emphasis is on treating the symptoms rather than the cause of the problem, e.g. a patient with spatial relations and body-image problems will have difficulty dressing him/herself; with practise, the patient will learn to dress but will still have the spatial relations and body-image problems. This approach is favoured by occupational therapists as it is more practical and more understandable to the patient. Patients often object to abstract perceptual training, finding it childish, degrading and irrelevant to their problems. The functional approach can be divided into two aspects: (a) compensation, where the patient is made aware of his/her problems and then taught to compensate or make allowances for them; and (b) adaptation, where the environment of the patient is changed to help the patient compensate for his/her symptoms.

Definitions of perceptual deficits and some treatment ideas (Edmans, 1987)

Body image and body schema

1. Body image: the visual and mental image of one's body (the feelings and thoughts rather than the exact picture of physical structure);

2. Body schema: how the patient perceives the position of the body and the relationships between the body parts (the patient needs to know this in order to know what, where and how to move);

3. Somatognosia: the lack of awareness of body structure and relationships, causing the patient to confuse sides of the body and body parts;

4. Unilateral neglect: the patient ignores one side of the body or environment;

5. Anosognosia: the patient fails to recognize the presence or the severity of the paralysis and denies the illness;

6. Right/left discrimination: the patient is unable to understand the concept of right and left.

In treating this type of perceptual disorder, a correct sitting and standing posture should be encouraged at all times. Use of the symmetrical approach (encouraging use of both halves of the body, e.g. the Bobath technique) will ensure the patient is aware of his whole body. Use of a mirror, particularly during dressing activities can often assist a patient to be aware of the affected side. Verbal cues may also be given during these activities. With walking practice, tape or footprints placed on the floor in a straight line or turning to the affected side can be followed by the patient. With transfers it is safer to teach the patients systematically so that they will carry them out exactly the same way each time. Right and left sides should be stressed during activities of daily living, cues such as 'your ring is on your left hand' and 'your watch is on your right wrist' can be given to the patient. It may help to mark the patient's clothes in some way, for example, a different coloured mark made on the left and right sleeves on clothing.

Spatial relationships

1. Figure ground: difficulty experienced in distinguishing the foreground from the background, for example, finding a brush in a cluttered draw, or the sleeve of a plain shirt;

2. Form constancy: inability to attend to subtle variations of form;

3. Position in space: the patient is unable to understand the concept of in/out, front/behind and up/down;

4. Spatial relations: the difficulty in perceiving the position of two or more objects in relation to him/herself or each other;

5. Topographical disorientation: difficulty in understanding and remembering relationships of places to one another, for example, finding the way between hospital buildings;
6. Depth and distance: the patient misjudges depth and distance, for example, has difficulty navigating stairs or continues to fill cups when they are full.

For re-education of figure ground, an article familiar to the patient should be placed on a table against a clear background, i.e. a background without any detail. A bright light should be shined onto the object and the patient told what the object is, it's shape, size, colour and uses, if any. Another object should then be added, preferably one that is related to the first, for example, a knife, plate and cup. The patient should be asked to pick up one of the objects named by the therapist. When the patient has become successful, other simple objects can be added, some relating to the first, others having no relationship whatsoever.

Another exercise that can be used is to introduce the patient to wooden shapes such as circles, squares and triangles. The patient should have the opportunity to feel the shapes in turn before moving on to the following exercise: a series of drawn shapes (e.g. a square with a circle partly covering it) should be shown to the patient. He/she should be asked to outline one of the shapes. When the patient has been successful, more complex tasks involving more shapes can be attempted.

For re-education of form-constancy, sets of the same shape in different sizes and thicknesses should be presented to the patient for sorting. To increase complexity, different shapes and colours can be added to the task. The shapes should then be related with the patient to everyday objects in the environment, e.g. a round clock on the wall related to a circle.

For re-education of position in space, the patient should be seated in front of a mirror with the therapist standing behind and asked to copy the therapist's movements. The patient can then be asked to touch parts of his/her body and to then touch the same part on the therapist's body by copying actions and verbal instructions. The next step is for the patient to touch a part of his/her body by instruction only. All types of movement should be experimented with until the patient has established his/her own awareness and that of other people. This can be reinforced with the use of jigsaw puzzles of people or body parts, doll dressing or during dressing practice.

Re-education of spatial relationships can best be achieved during feeding activities. Some patients have difficulty in seeing all of the items of food on a plate. In this case pictures can be related to objects before mealtimes to reinforce the relationships between the plate, the food and the cutlery used to eat it.

Apraxias

1. Constructional apraxia: inability to copy, draw or construct in 2–D or 3–D. This limits the patient's ability to perform purposeful acts while using objects in the environment;
2. Dressing apraxia: inability of the patient to dress because of a disorder of body schema and/or spatial relations;
3. Motor apraxia: loss of memory patterns resulting in the inability to perform purposeful tasks on command even though the patient understands the concepts and purpose of the task;
4. Ideomotor apraxia: inability to imitate gestures or perform purposeful motor tasks on command although the patient retains memory patterns and the ability to carry out old habitual tasks, for example, if a patient is asked to write with a pencil, he/she could describe the act and recognize it but not do it, yet at other times could write spontaneously;
5. Ideational apraxia: the patient can no longer carry out an act because he/she doesn't understand the concept or sequencing of the act, for example, when given a toothbrush and toothpaste the patient is unable to describe the functions of the items.

The main method of re-education of all apraxias is the perseverence in the practise of all activities in daily living, especially eating and dressing (i.e. activities requiring manipulation of objects and relating items in the environment to one's self).

Agnosias This is the lack of recognition of familiar objects perceived by the senses, i.e. visual, tactile, proprioceptive or auditory. Examples of agnosia are:

1. Visual object agnosia: inability to recognize objects even though visual activity and recognition of objects by touch are intact. Examples of this are: (a) simultanognosia: where the patient absorbs only one aspect of the whole picture; (b)

prospagnosia: the inability to recognize differences in faces; (c) colour agnosia: the inability to recognize colours; and (d) metamorphosia: where the objects appear bigger or smaller than they actually are;

2. Visual/spatial agnosia: a deficit in perceiving spatial relationships between objects or between objects and one's self, independently of visual object agnosia. This includes spatial relations, spatial orientation, topographical orientation, memory, and depth and distance;

3. Tactile agnosia: otherwise known as astereognosis, is the inability to recognize objects by handling when tactile, thermal and proprioceptive functions are intact.

As with apraxias, re-education in the above deficits takes place throughout the treatment-process mainly during activities of daily living. Specific tests and tasks are available and have been described in Chapter 2, page 28 (Assessment).

Assist in resettlement

Employment

If the patient is employed contact should be made with the employer as soon as possible to ascertain the situation regarding his/her return to work. If possible a fairly detailed description should be taken of the requirements of the job in order to assess whether the patient is likely to be able to return. It may be necessary to liaise with the employer on several occasions, perhaps to arrange a trial period at work or to discuss the possibility of reinstating the patient in a job where the activities are more suited to any residual disability. A work assessment should be set up and carried out at the appropriate time using simulated (or real) work activities of the particular type carried out at the patient's workplace.

A Disablement Resettlement Officer (DRO) may be contacted to assist with the process of resettlement or to arrange re-training in a new area of work. They are usually placed at Job Centres, and keep all the information about any employment opportunities available. When the patient returns to work (perhaps initially part-time) contact with the patient remains with the DRO, although the therapist may retain contact if the patient still attends the Out-patient's Department.

Acceptance of residual disability and the possibility that return to work may not be possible will be a devastating realization for the patient. Continuing support for both the patient and family during this time (possibly near the end of what may have been a long period of illness and rehabilitation) is especially necessary.

Leisure

Leisure and social activities can play an important part in the overall rehabilitation process, whether a patient returns to work or not. Many patients will return to participate in previous social activities and hobbies and where possible this should be encouraged. Any modification to techniques, tools or equipment can usually be devised, for example, adaptations to gardening tools, playing-card holders, etc. A wide variety of suggestions and ideas can be gained from visiting local centres such as the Red Cross or Disabled Living Centres. These centres keep a display and information on all aspects of disability and leisure pursuits.

USE OF COMPUTERS IN OCCUPATIONAL THERAPY DEPARTMENTS

Computers, in particular micro- or personal computers are playing an increasingly important role in occupational therapy departments throughout Great Britain and the United States. Computers can be very effective tools for the therapist to use and as therapists gain experience in using them they may well wish to use more specialized hardware and even program the computers themselves. In this way computers have become an invaluable aid in occupational therapy for stroke patients.

Arcade games

These are basically reaction games and are therefore of particular use for stroke rehabilitation. In playing these games the patient benefits by improving reaction times, generally improving in speed of thought processes, identifying possible perceptual problems and any difficulties in hand-eye co-ordination. However, most commercially available games are difficult to adapt to the intricacies and individual requirements of patients and therefore should be used discriminately.

Microcomputers in rehabilitation departments

The clinical use of microcomputers is well documented in the clinical psychology and rehabilitation literature (Skilbeck, 1984; Smart, 1988; Towle, Edmans and Lincoln, 1988), and in that of occupational therapy (Johnson and Garvie, 1985). Such uses have included the involvement of microcomputers in the measurement of sensory-motor function in a computerized preview tracking task (Jones and Donaldson, 1981) and in the evaluation of abnormal locomotion arising from stroke (Dzierzanowski *et al.*, 1985). However, the recognition and development of such applications was not seen until the late 1980s when researchers began to address other important areas in the rehabilitation of stroke. In addition to diagnosis and assessment, treatment and prognosis were included. Examples of these applications are: Thompson (1987c,d) for the use of microcomputers in the assessment and treatment of stroke; Hards, Thompson and Bate (1986) and Thompson, Hards and Bate (1986) for the treatment of hand and arm function using a microcomputer; Thompson (1984a) and McSherry and Fullerton (1985) for the use of computers in the prognosis of stroke.

As Hume (1984) suggested microcomputers have a definite therapeutic application in occupational therapy. Therapists have been slow to recognize the role of microcomputers possibly because of the unwillingness to accept new technology generally but more likely because of the need for therapist-programmers. This picture changed towards the end of the 1980s with therapists becoming increasingly involved both in adapting commercially-available programs and with writing programs for use in therapy. It is envisaged that computerized medical decision-making (Reggia, 1982) and expert systems (Tuhrim and Reggia, 1986; Thompson, 1987a) will be commonplace in most rehabilitation departments by the end of the century.

An example of the successful use of microcomputers in the treatment of stroke can be found in the Stroke Unit of City Hospital, Nottingham (Edmans 1987). Their aims of treatment when using the microcomputers are:

1. To improve perceptual deficits such as spatial relationships, inattention, scanning, sequencing and form constancy;
2. To improve visual comprehension;
3. To improve concentration;

4. To improve memory;
5. To improve co-ordination;
6. To provide mental stimulation.

To achieve this, a BBC B microcomputer with either a normal keyboard or a Microvitec touch-screen is used, with the occasional use of a concept keyboard. The software is usually purpose-written such as the Locheesoft OT/Remedial Software Series.

In general the patient does not use the computer directly. Instead, he/she sits upright at the table and lets the therapist operate the computer. In this way the patient concentrates on the task on the computer (the treatment is the task not whether the patient can operate the computer). However, when the touch screen is used the patient uses his/her unaffected hand to operate the computer with the affected limb in a reflex-inhibiting position. When the patient regains function in the affected upper limb this is used instead. Eventually the patient may be encouraged to use the ordinary keyboard using both affected and unaffected upper limbs.

All patients in the 15-bed unit use the computer as part of their treatment (this includes patients of all ages and all types of stroke). The choice of task depends on the severity of the stroke and the individual problems of each patient. For example a 76-year-old male with severe left hemiplegia and severe perceptual deficits, poor concentration and poor memory used the touch screen and remedial games to improve form constancy, spatial relationships, inattention, sequencing, concentration and memory. In another example, a 67-year-old male with right hemiplegia, receptive and expressive dysphasia (but no perceptual deficits) used the touch screen and Locheesoft therapy games for mental stimulation and improvement of concentration. Finally, a 21-year-old female with right hemiplegia, severe receptive and expressive dysphasia and spatial deficits used various remedial games for mental stimulation and improvement of spatial relationships.

Specialized hardware

A number of microcomputer peripherals have appeared on the market in response to the growing needs from the rehabilitation professions. These peripherals can usually be connected directly to the computer using user-ports or disk-drive sockets. Commercially available peripherals include the following:

1. Sculptured keyboard for use by the patient with limited finger movement (e.g. Maltron keyboard);
2. Redefinable keyboard with a flat area of definable keys/areas (e.g. concept keyboard);
3. Talking boxes comprizing simulated speech for use in speech therapy (e.g. Queenwood scientific talking box);
4. Spectacle frame with an infra-red sensor used to monitor eye position (e.g. Queenwood eye switch);
5. Touch sensitive surface and visual-display unit on which messages can be written by drawing each letter with a finger (e.g. Queenwood finger writer);
6. Touch screen (e.g.Microvitec 501);
7. Sensor which responds to vague and random limb movements of the user (e.g. Queenwood motion sensor);
8. Large rugged joystick incorporating microswitches (e.g. Voltmace delta handset);
9. Fine movement joystick (e.g. BBC Acorn joystick);
10. On-off tilt switch for forearm movement simulation (e.g. Queenwood tilt switch);
11. Foot-operated tilt switch (e.g. Cook Mercury tilt switch);
12. Shadow sensor responding to passage of shadow over sensitive area (e.g. Queenwood battery-powered shadow sensing switch);
13. Head-mounted torches worn on a headband detected by sensors to select/activate switches (e.g. Queenwood head torch, Queenwood gaze communication);
14. Rugged levers for mounting on the chest and activated by movement of the chin (e.g. Queenwood chin lever switch);
15. Head cradle-mounted switches operated by rotation of the head to the left and to the right (e.g. Queenwood head rotation switch);
16. Mouth-piece incorporating puff and suck switching elements (e.g. Queenwood puff and suck switch);
17. Pneumatic and electronic grip switches (e.g. Queenwood stretch sensitive switch);
18. Stretch sensor to monitor limb and trunk position (e.g. Queenwood stretch sensitive switch);
19. Hand held reaction time switch and software to measure manual dexterity (e.g. Paramedical Computing Thompson Reaction Time Switch – Thompson, 1987a);
20. Switch mounted on lower lip to detect if mouth is open or closed (e.g. Queenwood lip seal switch);

21. Versatile speech switches which produce authentic vocal sounds (e.g. Queenwood speech incentive sound switch);
22. Switch and software which detects muscular contraction and relaxation of leg muscles for improving control and testing reactions (e.g. Thompson Digital Switch – Thompson and Coleman, 1987d);
23. Adapted calculating and message writing devices (e.g. Queenwood memo communicator).

A comparison of input devices used with stroke patients was made by Petherham (1988). Five of the commonly available input devices were evaluated in tests undertaken by a number of stroke patients, in addition to a control group. The results showed that the tracker ball input device was most acceptable and gave rise to the highest success rates in the tests. The joystick and concept keyboard were rated next in line.

In order to use any peripherals, suitable software must exist in the computer, and sometimes this may be quite elaborate and complicated. It has often been debated whether or not occupational therapists should be trained, either during their normal patient contact hours or through attending short evening courses in computer literacy and familiarization. Some members of the profession have argued that the role of the OT does not include computer programming, while others hold the view that it is indeed the role of the modern-day OT to be able to include computing skills in therapy sessions. The debate is as yet unresolved with most schools of occupational therapy giving students only limited exposure to computing. However some schools recognize the growing need for computer awareness and have introduced keyboard skills, a basic understanding of the workings of a computer and evaluation of software into the teaching curriculum (Thompson and Morgan, 1989). In hospitals, some more progressive departments e.g. medical physics departments, either draw on local expertise to write programs for use in OT departments, or train OT to program microcomputers themselves. Some hospitals such as Stoke Mandeville, Aylesbury; Odstock Rehabilitation Unit, Salisbury and the Stroke Unit, Nottingham already make extensive use of computers and are involved in the development of peripherals and computer software.

Programming computers using Microtext

As mentioned in 'arcade games' (page 116) each patient has differing treatment needs and this requires flexibility from a computer. Unfortunately most commercially-written programs do not have this flexibility. Therefore in order to meet the needs of a particular patient or group of patients, the therapist needs to be able to program a computer him/herself. To do this, a simple dialogue programming language has been developed called Microtext.

Microtext enables non-programmers to write simple frame-by-frame programs for use in a number of different teaching or therapeutic settings and as such, is increasingly being used in occupational therapy departments in both Great Britain and the United States. Microtext uses the concept of a dialogue between the computer and the patient (described by Birnbaum, 1984). This involves a 'to and fro' movement of information from the user to the computer and back again. Typically the user sends a message to the computer, the computer analyses this and responds accordingly – the response usually involves transmitting a feedback message to the user. Information-exchange continues in this way until one or other of the communicating partners terminates the dialogue.

Microtext programs, therefore, are written as a series of frames. Each frame contains text for display to the user, response and branch instructions for the computer and general run-time commands. In this way dialogues can be built up that are tailored specifically for the patient by the therapist, without the therapist needing too much computer expertise.

Birnbaum (1984) reviewed the Microtext system and compared it with the conventional BBC BASIC (the computer language supplied with the popular BBC microcomputer). Microtext is frame-oriented (in a sense very much like viewdata systems such as TELETEXT) and yet each frame contains control information integral to each frame. In this way Microtext combines the ease of use of viewdata with the flexibilities of a programming language. For the non-programmer, Microtext offers a wide variety of facilities that are relatively simple to use. But for the confident and competent programmer, BASIC still has a considerably greater range of facilities than Microtext.

FURTHER READING

The following cover all areas of the treatment of stroke:

Coleman, M.J. (1984) *Disk Programming Techniques for the BBC Microcomputer,* Prentice-Hall International, London.

Coll, J. (1982) *The BBC Microcomputer Guide,* British Broadcasting Corporation, London.

Davies, P.M. (1985) *Steps to Follow: A Guide to the Treatment of Adult Hemiplegia,* Springer-Verlag, New York.

Department of Health and Social Security, *Handbook of Wheelchairs and Bicycles and Tricycles,* MHM 408, London.

Edmans, J. (1987), *Handbook for the Rehabilitation of Stroke Patients,* The occupational therapy department, General Hospital, Nottingham.

Edmans, J.A. and Lincoln, N.B. (1987) The frequency of perceptual deficits after stroke, *Clinical Rehabilitation,* **1,** 273–81.

Eggers, O. (1983) *Occupational Therapy in the Treatment of Adult Hemiplegia,* Heinemann , London.

Petherham, B. (1988) Enabling stroke victims to interact with a computer – a comparison of input devices, *International Disability Studies,* **10,** 73–80.

Sime, M.S. and Coombes, M.J. (1983) *Designing for Human – Computer Communication,* Academic Press, London.

Simpson, R.J. (1987) Remedial therapy referral times for stroke patients, *British Journal of Occupational Therapy,* **50,** 11, 379–80.

Smart, S. (1988) Computers as treatment: The use of the computer as an occupational therapy medium, *Clinical Rehabilitation,* **2,** 61–9.

Sunderland, A., Wade, D.T., and Hewer, R.L. (1987) The natural history of visual neglect after stroke, *International Disability Studies,* **9,** 55–9.

Thompson, S.B.N. and Coleman, M.J. (1987) Leg-injured patients switch on to rehabilitation, *Therapy Weekly,* **13,** 48, 7.

Towle, D., Edmans, J.A. and Lincoln, N.B. (1988) Use of computer-presented games with memory-impaired stroke patients, *Clinical Rehabilitation,* **2,** 303–7.

Trombley, C.A. (ed.) (1983) *Occupational Therapy for Physical Dysfunction,* 2nd edn, Williams and Wilkins, Baltimore.

Turner, A. (ed.) (1987) *The Practice of Occupational Therapy,* 2nd edn, chs 13, 18, Churchill Livingstone, London.

Examples of suitable software used at the Stroke Unit, Nottingham

BN 1, 2, 3 and 4, Burden Neurological Institute, Bristol.

Dorset 4, obtained from Derby School of Occupational Therapy.

Locheesoft Publications; available from Locheesoft Publications Ltd, Oak Villa, New Alyth, Blairgowrie PH11, Scotland.

USA disk, obtained from Nether Edge Hospital, Sheffield.

5

Biofeedback in Rehabilitation

The modern interpretation of biofeedback is the technique of using electronic equipment to reveal instantaneously to patients and therapists particular physiological events and to teach the patients to control these otherwise involuntary events by manipulating the displayed signals (usually visual and/or acoustic). As it is now being practised, biofeedback is a scientific technique rather than a separate science but the basic concept has stimulated the beginnings of a probable revolution in medical science which encompasses both medical and paramedical approaches. This new approach is often termed behavioural medicine.

The use of behavioural techniques is emphasized in behavioural medicine and has been used for the treatment of a host of disturbances, ranging from recurring headaches (Johnson and Turin, 1975) to severe cardiovascular problems (Basmajian, 1981). Patients with physical handicaps of varying degrees have been sharing the benefits of biofeedback techniques for some time now but it is only recently, with the advent of microcomputer technology, that the range of benefit is being assessed.

Biofeedback techniques have matured considerably since their conception in the 1960s. The history of biofeedback can be traced to the formation of a small society; the Biofeedback Research Society in Santa Monica, California, in 1969 (Basmajian, 1981). A group of investigators, who recognized a common theme of study met to discuss biological feedback mechanisms in psychotherapy. The common theme had grown from a number of studies which demonstrated the human capacity to alter normally unconscious physiological activities while being monitored by electronic diagnostic devices. By concentrating on increasing or decreasing the electronic signals indicating the level of physiological activity a person could alter many processes in the body which are not normally felt or sensed in any way.

Three main scientific sources can be identified as being the broadstream of modern biofeedback: (a) electromyography (EMG); (b) electroencephalography (EEG); (c) cardiovascular physiology. Electromyography is the continuous recording of the electrical activity of a muscle by means of electrodes inserted into or placed onto the muscle fibres. The tracing is displayed on an oscilloscope. Electroencephalography is the technique for recording the electrical activity from different parts of the brain and cardiovascular physiology is the study of the behaviour of the heart with particular interest in the vessels both within the heart and those that supply it with blood. Feedback applications within this area have included attempts at reducing blood pressure levels in patients with high blood pressure. Other types of feedback include visual and acoustic which will be discussed further.

ELECTROMYOGRAPHY

It is interesting to note that despite the recognition of the considerable assistance derived from the instant feedback of myoelectric signals the use of biofeedback techniques for the rehabilitation of patients is a fairly recent application and that only two studies made reference to the clinical possibilities of EMG before the 1960s (Mims, 1956; Marinacci and Horande, 1960).

However, several studies in the late 1950s and early 1960s were exploring the possibilities of employing feedback signals to train specific controls in normal muscles of handicapped persons to substitute for lost limbs (Basmajian, 1963). One important study by Basmajian (1967) sought to determine and define the normal mechanisms of motor control in various parts of the body and developed methods for treating neurologically and orthopaedically handicapped patients. By the late 1960s there was a worldwide movement for the development and use of electrically activated artificial limbs and the need for scientific understanding was of paramount importance.

In the midst of these studies it was found that subjects provided with instant visual and acoustic feedback of the EMG signals arising from invisible and unfelt contractions of their muscles could learn to perform elaborate tricks with the tiniest units of muscle – the motor units (Basmajian, 1981). Since each motor unit is supplied by a single motor neurone, it became obvious that patients were being trained to achieve conscious control of individual motor cells in the spinal cord: a phenomenon then considered by most neurologists to be impossible. Perhaps more importantly it was also discovered that subjects could put a single cell through elaborate skills while completely inhibiting the activity of the surrounding cells. Subjects could consciously relax all the muscle fibres in a muscle (or even a whole limb) while activating the target motor unit in isolation.

As Basmajian (1981) points out, not only can patients fire single motor cells with an active suppression or inhibition of neighbouring cells, but they can also produce deliberate changes in the rate of firing. Most people can do this if they are provided with aural or visual cues from their muscles by EMG. Descriptions of a typical training procedure are well known. Following the implantation of special fine-wired electrodes in any voluntary skeletal muscle, a patient needs to be given only general instruction.

The patient is asked to make contractions of the muscle under study while listening to and seeing the motor-unit potentials on the monitors. A typical period of up to 15 minutes is sufficient to familiarize him/her with the response of the apparatus to a range of movements and postures. Patients are invariably amazed at the responsiveness of the loudspeaker and cathode ray tube to their slightest efforts and they accept these without difficulty as a new form of internal body awareness or artificial proprioception (Basmajian, 1981).

VISUAL FEEDBACK

One combination of biofeedback techniques commonly used experimentally is EMG and visual feedback (Amato, Hermsmeyer and Kleinman, 1973). In this situation a visual display may be connected to the electromyograph so that the patient can be given a visual indication of neuromuscular performance via a visual-display unit. Using a graphics monitor, a pictoral display, histograms, pie charts or graphs may be constructed and displayed in place of a standard cathode ray oscilloscope, potentially providing the patient with a whole range of visual indicators and incentives. Similarly, an auditory feedback mechanism can be established by issuing a tone in place of a changing visual display.

In a study by Bazzini et al. (1984), both sides of a hemiplegic group of patients were assessed and treated using a visual feedback technique. Evaluation of a specific group of muscles (with and without the aid of visual feedback) was carried out. A visual display provided patients with a graphical indication of their performance and a hardcopy polygraph record was also generated for later analysis. In this study a marked increase was noted in the muscular contractions of the hemiplegic side (Bazzini *et al.*, 1984). This is one typical application in which visual feedback has been used as an indicator of patients' performance. Visual displays can also be useful to the therapist in providing an instantaneous indication of muscular contraction, skin response, or limb movement. Indeed the scope for its use is great and with the potential capabilities of microcomputer technology, visual feedback is playing an increasingly important role in biofeedback techniques. Technology has also progressed in the range of feedback facilities available. Use of portable biotechnological feedback devices in systems of active rehabilitative therapy are growing in popularity (Demidenko *et al.*, 1983), whether acoustic (Brzoza, Janota and Wolniczek, 1981; Gruskin, Abitante and Gorski, 1983), or visual (Alexander, French and Goodman, 1975).

A typical visual display may comprise a moving oscilloscope-beam representing the electrical activity of a chosen muscle group, or alternatively a graphical display consisting of a moving line or histogram to indicate the level of activity reached during a therapy session.

In the early 1980s there was little ingenuity in the variety of visual displays used during feedback. Simplicity is an important consideration when designing a display, though this has tended in the past to lead towards a narrow choice of unexciting and perhaps oversimplified displays. The origin may lie in the problems involved in interfacing equipment. Previous applications of graphics have been in connection with EMG treatment, where information concerning neuromuscular activity is communicated using a moving oscilloscope-beam representing the electrical activity of muscles during certain rehabilitative exercises. In order to enhance the display more versatile equipment, such as a microcomputer and a colour monitor may be interfaced with the electromyograph. A changing raster graphics display, similar to a TV picture, is potentially much more motivating than a thin moving line.

Visual displays have been used in a number of different treatment applications. Davis and Lee (1980) have used a vector display (solid line) as an aid for co-ordinating activity in antagonistic muscle groups. Patients using this therapy were able to modify the patterns of EMG activity in antagonistic muscles by using the visual feedback information concerning relative activation of certain muscle groups. Patients suffering from either hemiplegia or cerebellar inco-ordination were also able to utilize the feedback to reduce the amount of inappropriate coactivation of flexors and extensors and to produce more sustained and regular activation of individual muscle groups during a simple wrist flexion-extension task.

The effect of the biofeedback was found to be almost immediate in some patients and particularly in the hemiplegics. They were able to modify their EMG pattern at the first biofeedback session, and over a period of time they were able to maintain this change independent of feedback (Davis and Lee, 1980).

Several questions must be considered before determining whether such results justify a more extensive trial of EMG biofeedback of the type discussed. First, was the apparent improvement in EMG activation directly related to the information provided by biofeedback or could it have been due to associated factors? The exposure to rather complex electronic equipment was a novel experience for the patients and might have conceivably introduced a placebo effect. The attention focused on the patient and his/her hemiplegic arm might also have led to an increased level of motivation which could have produced the results observed.

However, several factors suggest that the changes observed with biofeedback were more than a non-specific placebo effect. The patients studied had stable motor deficits which had not changed for several months despite prolonged periods of conventional therapy. Also one patient was not able to perform so well when provided with 'distorted' feedback, suggesting that the alteration in EMG pattern occurring with feedback was due to the specific information contained in the true feedback signal. However, it is not clear from this study exactly what was presented to the patient during a 'distorted' feedback session.

Clearly, if this approach is going to be of practical value in rehabilitation of patients with motor deficits such as stroke, it must be shown that improved patterns of motor activity which develop during visual feedback can be transferred to everyday tasks. Preliminary work has already begun to develop a battery of functional tests to provide a quantitative assessment of upper-extremity motor control (Davis and Lee, 1980; Thompson, Hards and Bate,

1986; Thompson, 1987a) and such an assessment for lower-limb extremity motor control has also proved highly successful (Thompson, 1987b,c; Thompson and Coleman 1987a).

AUDITORY FEEDBACK

Auditory feedback techniques have included the presentation of white noise to one of the patient's ears while the patient attends to a simple auditory task with the other ear. Correct responses to an auditory task may be indicated by interrupting the attended message, or by breaking the continuity in the transmission of white noise.

Visual and auditory feedback techniques have also been used in combination with positional feedback stimulation as a treatment for facilitating knee extension (Winchester *et al.*, 1983) and ankle dorsiflexion (Johnson and Garton, 1973), and generally for gait training (Koheil and Mandel, 1980). Stimulation-training provides the patient with immediate auditory and visual feedback of the changing joint angle whilst voluntarily extending the limb. When the patient reaches a near maximum extension effort, electrical stimulation of the muscle group is automatically triggered, completing the patient's available range of movement (ROM) in extension. Winchester and colleagues suggested that positional-feedback-stimulation training is especially effective when used to augment a facilitation programme for improving knee extension control in hemiparetic patients (Winchester *et al.*, 1983) and apparently works well in the auditory-visual combination which has been implemented.

COMPARISON OF VISUAL AND AUDITORY FEEDBACK

The role of biofeedback in reducing abnormal muscle tone has been well documented for several years but the particular type of feedback to be used in various situations still provides debate among researchers and clinicians. Comparing auditory, visual and tactile methods for producing reduced muscle activity (Schandler and Grings, 1976) it was found that auditory feedback showed significant reductions after treatment on all measures, i.e. heart rate, systolic blood pressure, respiration rate, extensor EMG, and frontalis (muscle of forehead) EMG. While producing significant reductions in heart rate, respiratory rate and EMG activity, the visual feedback showed EMG post-treatment levels above post-treatment tactile feedback. Furthermore, Alexander, French and Goodman (1975) showed that auditory EMG feedback from the frontalis muscle led subjects to decrease frontalis activity significantly, while visual EMG feedback from the frontalis was ineffective. Other researchers have noted no difference between activity and visual feedback in the self-control of heart rate (Blanchard and Young, 1972).

The characteristics of EMG biofeedback have often shown rapid effects after minimal training and high subjective involvement (Gaudette, Prins and Kahane, 1983). It is possible to conclude that EMG feedback procedures may well be suited for reducing psychological and physiological correlates of tension during relatively short-term laboratory sessions. Researchers have subsequently concentrated their efforts towards determining the short-term and significant superiority of either auditory or visual EMG feedback in the reduction of frontal (i.e. forehead) muscle activity. However, as many reports have shown, there are several confounding factors in determining this significance: for example, the orbiculoris oculi muscle which surrounds the eye is more relaxed when the eye is closed, allowing the frontal muscle to be more relaxed. Hence, for feedback to be effective in reducing frontal muscle activity, the patient's eyes must be closed, thus denying the possibilities of improvement associated with visual feedback techniques.

Thompson (1984a, 1985a) and Thompson and Coleman (1987b) have shown that visual and auditory feedback can be effective in producing improved reaction times in the quadriceps muscles of hemiparetic and hemiplegic patients. Significant evidence was found after a three-week period to suggest that there was a decrease in muscular reaction times (i.e. an improvement) after using computer-assisted visual feedback. However, it is speculative as to whether or not muscle tonus returned naturally and that feedback was useful solely as an assessment tool at this stage in treatment, or alternatively, that continuous testing using visual feedback had made return of function in the lower limbs more rapid. However, it can be said of visual feedback that it is an attractive and increasingly more accepted approach to the treatment of head injury and that there is growing interest within the paramedical professions for its use in the treatment of stroke victims.

129

FEEDBACK INDUCED MUSCULAR EXERCISE

In this procedure the elbow on the paretic side is coupled to the shaft of a specially designed electric motor. A signal corresponding to the velocity of movement is amplified and applied to the power amplifier supplying the motor. The sense of the connection is such as to provide positive velocity feedback (Gelman *et al.*, 1978); thus a force is provided which assists the limb in its motion. With high gain the system is unstable and oscillates at a rate which depends on the inertia of the limb and the mechanical and reflex behaviour of the musculature. The stiffer the limb, the higher the rate of the oscillations and the smaller the amplitude.

The patient's arm is always bandaged to the splint before power is applied. The force available from the motor is dependent on current-limiting in the power amplifier. This value is adjusted for each patient so as to give a wide range of motion: the stiffer the limb, the more the force that is needed.

Gelman *et al.* (1978) assessed the value of this exercise in the treatment of stroke patients using daily periods of exercise of up to 20 minutes. Mobilization of the joints is considered to be an essential element in the therapy of stroke patients and it is generally accepted that in the occupational therapist's treatment of paresis; passive movements may be desirable, and often even necessary, to prevent shortening of joint capsules, ligaments and muscles. In addition passive movements may possibly help the patient to relearn the use of his/her muscles. The limb motion is in the horizontal plane and voluntary motion can thus easily be appreciated by the patient at a stage when it is essentially absent when contending with gravity. There is an interaction between the person and the machine which the more curious and intellectually preserved patient will find interesting. With such a machine it is feasible to provide movements for longer periods than would be practical for an occupational therapist to spend with one patient.

JOINT POSITION FEEDBACK

Genu recurvatum (full extension or hyperextension of the knee during the stance phase of gait) is one of the major causes of disturbance in the walking pattern of stroke patients. This gait dysfunction is often due to the failure of the quadriceps muscles to cease contracting at the proper time (Koheil and Mandel, 1980).

Normal gait patterns have been thoroughly studied (Wall and Ashburn, 1979) and analysed by electromyography and electrogoniometry. Early and mid-stance phases of normal gait produce an extension-flexion-extension (E-F-E) action at the knee joint. That is, at heel strike, the knee is fully extended or nearly so; then knee flexion of short duration and small range occurs as a result of the body weight coming over the foot. This short period of flexion is then followed by extension of the knee. The foregoing actions facilitate a smooth forward movement of the body. However, in many stroke patients this normal E-F-E pattern is disrupted. Weight-bearing usually elicits a contraction in the quadriceps muscle group but these muscles do not regulate their function in accordance with the normal gait pattern and thus hyperextension of the knee often occurs when the E-F-E pattern should be present.

Occupational therapy pertaining to knee action during gait training in stroke patients is usually directed at promoting alternating action of knee flexor and extensor muscles. In most cases, special emphasis must be given to training the hamstring muscles (knee flexors). Patients who do not achieve this alternating muscle activity usually exhibit genu recurvatum varying from mild to severe (Koheil and Mandel, 1980). A hyperextended knee is stable and also a good compensatory action for patients unable to achieve proper knee control. However, achieving a normal gait pattern is desirable to avoid damage due to abnormal stresses on joint structures and to reduce the need for walking aids or splinting.

Biofeedback is a tool of growing importance in the field of stroke rehabilitation. While recognizing that the provision of immediate and accurate information about covert activity in the rehabilitation patient may substitute for inadequate proprioception, it may be used to facilitate greater accuracy in shaping patient responses, thus assisting both the therapist and patient in the total rehabilitative process.

Several studies have been published in which biofeedback was utilized in gait training with patients having suffered neurological damage (Fernando and Basmajian, 1978). Johnson and Garton (1973) used auditory and visual electromyographical feedback to treat ankle dorsiflexion paralysis (foot-drop) in ten hemiplegic patients who were at least one year post-stroke. Using a subjective rating scale for motor function all ten patients improved in muscle strength over the course of the study. Amato, Hermsmeyer and

Kleinman (1973) used visual electromyographical biofeedback to teach inhibition of spasticity in the gastrocnemius (calf) muscle of a young man nine years after he had suffered a severe stroke. They reported improvement in the patient's active range of ankle movement and in his muscle strength, with the generalized effect of improved gait.

Two foot-switches were used in conjunction with a tone avoidance procedure by Spearing and Poppen (1974) to reduce foot-dragging in an adult patient with cerebral palsy. Through specific placement of the switches on the client's shoe, the number of steps and foot drags which occurred during a session could be recorded on a counter worn on the patient's belt. Results indicated a dramatic decrease in foot-dragging with the contingent aversive feedback, with some deterioration during no-feedback trials and at a 3-month follow-up. The authors hypothesized that the feedback contingency may have indirectly provoked the client into stretching the tendons associated with the gastrocnemius-soleus muscles, thus accounting for the improvement. This procedure has distinct possibilities for a range of pareses, notably those caused by cerebral lesions as with the majority of stroke patients.

In an American study, Basmajian et al. (1975) attempted to compare the effectiveness of conventional physiotherapy (Group I) with conventional physiotherapy plus biofeedback (Group II) in the treatment of 20 adult hemiplegic patients with foot-drop. Strength of dorsiflexion, active range of motor and functional-gait improvement were the chosen parameters. The biofeedback group received both auditory and visual feedback. Change in strength and range of movement were almost twice as great in Group II as in Group I. Some patients in Group I did exhibit improvement and the authors suggested that biofeedback could have facilitated this potential. However, improvements in range of movement and maximum strength must be converted into functional change to be meaningful. At the conclusion of this study, three patients from Group II were able to walk without a short-leg brace. Feedback proved to be greatly motivating and was shown to be a useful tool in stroke rehabilitation.

Wolf, Baker and Kelly (1979) in the USA have shown that biofeedback training facilitates therapy in the training of stroke victims, including those of long-standing disability; and Koheil and Mandel (1980) have investigated the possibility of training a hemiplegic patient exhibiting genu recurvatum to maintain slight knee flexion at mid-stance so that extension did not exceed the neutral position. In this study, in addition to the clear improvement in her genu recurvatum, the patient was able to progress from quad stick to a standard walking stick. Clinically, the patient's gait became more stable without a sacrifice in the speed of gait. Although a 30° flexion angle was set to prevent excessive knee flexion as compensatory action while the patient was attempting to stop genu recurvatum, this limit was in fact never surpassed. In general, it appeared that the patient's performance varied with the state of her health and with her level of fatigue.

In an attempt to carry out a thorough assessment of the patient's gait, modelled after Ogg (1963), videotapes were analysed for information concerning step distance, stride length, foot placement angles and width of base. The changes noted were relatively consistent in each of the three treatment phases. There was an overall decrease in stride length and step distance. The walking base, in terms of distance between right and left heel placements, increased and the foot placement angles for both feet became slightly inverted from the initial placement measurements. Since these changes occured in each treatment phase it is difficult to derive definitive statements relating to their aetiology and importance. Recognizing that many changes did occur during the treatment session, it was suggested that a careful evaluation of other aspects of gait be made when practical.

The results of this particular study emphasize the potential usefulness of joint position biofeedback as part of the total therapeutic approach to gait training in hemiplegic patients. This also supports the findings of Basmajian et al. (1975) that biofeedback is a useful adjunct to therapy in stroke rehabilitation.

SENSOR PAD AND LIMB-LOAD MONITOR

A number of portable biotechnical devices have been used in the treatment of stroke patients (Demidenko et al., 1983). Most forms of biofeedback are expensive and it is often not realistic to use them as an everyday aid to treatment for large numbers of patients in an occupational therapy department. Sensor pads are one example of a relatively inexpensive aid that can provide auditory feedback during a typical therapy session (Triptree and Harrison, 1980).

Before the patient uses the sensor pad the therapist may ask him/her to perform the desired activity and so gauge the approximate pressure required. Throughout the activity performed by the patient, the sensitivity can be adjusted so that at first an audible signal is produced with only a slight transference of weight, the sensitivity of the pad being reduced as the patient improves and becomes able to transfer weight correctly. It has been found that patients become skilled in weight transference more quickly when auditory feedback of their progress is provided (Triptree and Harrison, 1980), although this is dependent on good auditory function of the patient.

Suitable positions for weight transference using the sensor pad include:

1. Patient lying prone with forearm support; large pad placed under affected elbow and forearm. Patient rocks his/her weight on to affected side to produce audible signal;
2. Patient sitting with large pad under affected buttock. Patient transfers weight on to affected side to produce audible signal;
3. Patient standing with or without support, small pad placed under heel of affected side, transfers weight from one foot to the other, producing audible signal each time weight is correctly transferred through affected leg.

A small heel-shaped sensor pad can be fitted into the patient's shoe; a battery box or amplifier is attached to the leg by a Velcro band. From simple weight transference the patient can then progress to maintaining weight through the affected side while performing a movement with the sound side or gross movement of the whole body.

A development of sensory feedback during weight-bearing activities has been the Limb Load Monitor (LLM) which consists of a force transducer housed within a footplate placed in the sole of a shoe (Kwatny and Zuckerman, 1975). The footplate is connected to the LLM by a coaxial cable. An audible tone can be emitted through an amplifier placed within the LLM when force upon the plate reaches a preset (threshold) value. Through training by shaping responses to attempts at symmetrical standing, some hemiplegic patients can correct their static limb loading patterns (Wannstedt and Herman, 1978) and possibly retain these corrected patterns once feedback has been withdrawn.

The LLM can be used either as a force-feedback device for weight-shifting during stance or by adding a time delay modification as incorporated in the modified Krusen LLM (Wolf and

Hudson, 1980), for feedback to the existing force-sensing component. The modified device can be used during walking activities by controlling two variables, force and time delay, over which a specified force is applied to the footplate to produce one auditory feedback tone during the stance phase of the gait cycle. This time delay addition is important because feedback information about stance phase of gait should depend not just upon force through the limb, but the time over which such force is exerted.

Although the LLM and modification have proven to be clinically effective, their precision as research and measurement tools has yet to be determined. For example, force distribution through the footplate must be compared to opposite forces on a force platform when the plate is worn either within or on the undersurface of a shoe. Measurements for accuracy of force transmission might be the next logical development for this device.

MICROCOMPUTER GRAPHICS IN FEEDBACK THERAPY

Probably the most significant modern clinical application of microcomputer graphics is with hemiplegic patients during rehabilitation (Bazzini *et al.*, 1984). The potential of computer-assisted feedback therapies has not been fully recognized, with many established therapies remaining denied of the range and versatility of computer technology. Such is the case with oscilloscope-based therapies like electromyography (Basmajian, 1981; Wolf and Binder-MacLeod, 1983).

During the past decade occupational therapists have become increasingly aware of the range of electronic aids and equipment available, particularly in relation to patients with mobility or communication problems. Power-assisted equipment for the severely handicapped is now in general use, and the developments in technology in its widest sense have forced the paramedical professions into considering the therapeutic potential of microcomputers in addition to, for example, videos and toys.

According to Hume (1984) considerable evidence of the application of microcomputers within education, communication and administration exists, but nothing in relation to therapy, assessment, or prognosis. Although this would seem rather an over-generalization, past literature does indicate a severe lack of clinical usage of microcomputer technology, especially in providing visual feedback during rehabilitation and assessment.

In an attempt to resolve this situation, a pilot study was conducted at the School of Information Science, Portsmouth Polytechnic, UK, to assess the usefulness of computer-assisted visual feedback on adult hemiparetics and hemiplegics (Thompson, 1984a). Patients from Queen Alexandra Hospital, Cosham, England, were tested over a six-week period for their reaction times to a changing graphics display. Two research hypotheses proposed that change in response time of the affected lower limb of a patient in the mid-stroke category was different to that of a patient in the late-stroke category.

There was no significant evidence (at 5% level – i.e. 95 times in 100 this was the case) to suggest that there was a difference between the muscular contraction times but significant evidence (at 2% level – i.e. 98 times in 100 this was the case) was found to suggest that change in quadriceps tendon and biceps femoris response times (i.e. muscular relaxation) of a patient in the mid-stroke category was higher than that of a patient in the late-stroke category. It was also shown that there was a significant improvement (at 2% level) in contraction times during weeks two and three of the study. These findings indicate the importance of computer-assisted visual feedback and quadriceps reaction times in providing a potential prognostic tool for adult hemiplegia in occupational therapy. The study also shows a promising new application of information systems within the paramedical professions.

In order to appreciate the potential of microcomputers used in this way, it is perhaps useful to briefly describe the patient's point of view of the computer-assisted therapy used in this study. Eight stages can be described which illustrate the changes in the graphics display. The session proceeds as follows (Thompson, Coleman and Yates, 1986):

1. The display screen initially shows a simple screen (Figure 5.1): an open drawbridge over a sea channel with a lorry waiting to cross the bridge. A prominent 'sun' is also displayed;
2. The therapy sequence begins with the computer emitting a cueing tone. The single note is a stimulus to the patient to exert pressure on a quadriceps switch by contraction of the quadriceps. In addition to the tone, a visual stimulus is given by means of the 'sun' disappearing;
3. Detection by the microcomputer of sufficient pressure on the quadriceps switch now causes the display to change, again in a clear but simple manner: the drawbridge closes (Figure 5.2);

Figure 5.1 No response display.

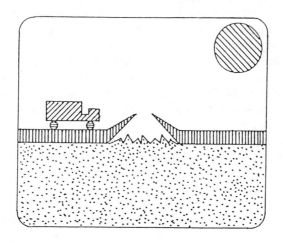

Figure 5.2 Response display.

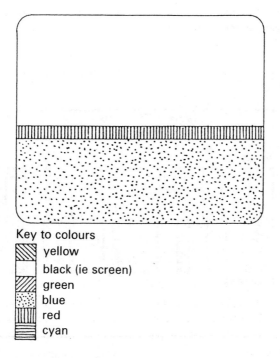

Key to colours
yellow
black (ie screen)
green
blue
red
cyan

4. The cueing tone is emitted continuously. During this time the patient will endeavour to maintain pressure on the quadriceps switch and the visual feedback will indicate that this is, or is not, being achieved. This immediately overcomes the difficulty faced by many hemiplegic patients in not knowing whether muscle contraction or relaxation has occurred;

5. When the tone stops the patient has to relax the thigh muscles (mainly the quadriceps tendon and rectus femoris). This is indicated by the visual display returning to its original 'open drawbridge';

6. Steps 1–5 are repeated a further eight times. The onset of the cueing tone is produced by the computer at varying intervals and is maintained for periods of varying length;

7. During the course of the whole exercise, the microcomputer also records two time lags; firstly, the time delay between the onset of the cueing tone and the subsequent detection of pressure on the quadriceps switch, and secondly the delay between the cessation of the cueing tone and relaxation on the quadriceps switch. These results are then displayed on the screen in the form of a bar chart (Figure 5.3);

8. By repeating the whole exercise for both affected and unaffected limbs, a comparison can be made of their respective performance.

Figure 5.3 Diagrammatic representation of computer screen results display.

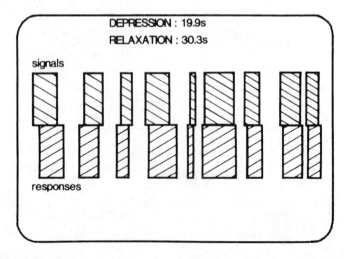

As with any experimental study there are inevitably a number of criticisms that can be made concerning the design or the findings of the study. When assessing the validity of such findings, consideration should be given to the apparatus itself. The quadriceps switch (QS) used in this study required considerable adjustment for each patient. The exact position of the pressure pad, above and behind the patella, may not always have been precisely matched for each patient. A jig to align this critical position may have reduced the inevitable errors involved.

Two switch positions were also discovered during the initial testing of the apparatus. The second lower 'click' activated the pressure pad: the first being an extra connection common to the standard switch component. Indeed, it served only as a potential inhibitor of task performance (Thompson, 1984a). In practice, although patients were aware of the two 'clicks', their concentration on the visual display was great enough for them to take note of the visual feedback (i.e. the closing bridge display) and to ignore the spurious first switch position of the QS. Since this is an integral component of the apparatus, it has the possibilities for future development. The switch position could provide an indication of the pressure applied to the pad (Thompson, 1987d; Thompson and Coleman, 1987c,d), or an alternative visual (or auditory) display. Certainly it was important to be aware of this feature in the event of mis-responding to the cueing tones.

Another feature that warrants discussion is the presentation of the display itself. In the Thompson (1984a) study there were three main visual displays: (i) an open drawbridge; (ii) a closed drawbridge; and (iii) a results screen. The first two screens can be regarded as 'patient' displays (i.e. providing the patient with information). They can also be considered as 'fun' displays in terms of giving the patient an incentive in order to maintain or increase his/her motivation towards operating the QS. The third display can be regarded as a 'therapist – scientific' display (i.e. this display was essentially for the therapist and provided scientific data for later comparison with other performances and with other similar patients).

It is difficult to decide whether or not a display should be solely for the patient or for the therapist. Clearly, if a therapy is to work successfully, the display should motivate the patient – hence a 'patient-fun' display should be used during the time when a response is required by the patient. However, when the results are to be displayed they should be presented in a way that is readily

139

understood by the patient (and thus motivate the patient by indicating an achievement) but should also provide meaningful, objective, scientific data for interpretation by the therapist.

Whether or not these two requirements can be met in a single display is dependent on the task being performed and on the measurements taken. For instance a numerical value may be meaningful to the therapist and may enable direct comparisons with other performances or with other patients, but remains apparently arbitrary and meaningless to the patient. Resolving this problem requires careful consideration of the specific task being measured; for the assessment battery used in the Thompson study (1987e), the primary concern was to provide the therapist with scientific data but, at the same time, it was important not to exclude the patient from the results by presenting a rather esoteric display.

In addition to these problems is the actual measurement to be taken of the patient's performance. In the study described previously a digital (on/off) signal from the QS was interpreted by the microcomputer and appropriate displays were presented. During other forms of measurement, for example, measuring the electrical activity of muscles using an electromyograph (Thompson, 1986; 1987d) an analogue signal may be produced. This is a continuous signal comprising a variation in the values of, for example, electrical voltage in the muscles as produced by nerve impulses. These changes in electrical activity are not simply one or two values, as with signals from the QS. Therefore, each signal detected must be given a bit value (i.e. 1 or 0) for interpretation by the microcomputer.

In effect, the analogue signal is converted to a series of digital signals which can be read by the microcomputer software – via the analogue port. A fast analogue-to-digital converter can be used to sample the input analogue signal from a device, such as an electromyograph, and converts each chosen sample to a digital value for presentation to the microcomputer. A piece of coding can then be used to interpret these digital values and subsequently draws out a series of graphics, or performs another operation such as providing performance information. Such methods for providing graphics displays from an input analogue signal via an electromyograph have been documented elsewhere (Thompson, 1986; 1987d, e).

MICROCOMPUTER-ASSISTED FEEDBACK THERAPY

Electromyographical treatment of stroke is well documented (Lee *et al.*, 1976; Mroczek, Halpern and McHugh, 1978; Marsh, 1980; Felsenthal, 1982a,b). Treatment by feedback induced muscular exercise is also well known (Vodovnik and Rebersek, 1973; Gelman *et al.*, 1978; Stanic *et al.*, 1978; Baker *et al.*, 1979). Integration of computers into therapies themselves has produced considerable interest among researchers (Cassell, Shaw and Stern, 1973; Doerr, Estes and Tourtellotte, 1977), and has included the use of microcomputers to provide graphic feedback displays (Jones, 1975) such as for use in visual feedback therapy (Thompson, 1984a; 1985b; Thompson, Coleman and Yates, 1986; Thompson, Hards and Bate, 1986), and as a controlled training aid for the handicapped (Thompson, 1986; Thompson 1987a; Thompson and Coleman, 1987d; Figure 5.4).

A preview tracking task has also been developed (Jones and Donaldson, 1981) which has particular application to neurological assessment and rehabilitation. Generated and monitored by a graphic display computer, it permits global quantification of the upper-limb sensory-motor system. The incorporation of 'preview' into visually tracking a 'circuit' is considered to significantly increase its effectiveness and relevance in relation to normal daily activities. Applied to brain-damaged patients, particularly head injury or stroke, the preview tracking task allows assessment at regular intervals enabling sensory-motor recovery curves to be generated. The potential of this technique, to help determine the efficiency of therapeutic procedures on the recovery process, is significantly useful when combined with a less frequently applied but more component-specific neurological assessment battery.

Although evaluation of the sensory and motor systems individually is reasonably straightforward in routine clinical neurological assessment, the same cannot be said for their integration in the performance of more complex tasks. Tracking tasks have become firmly established as one of the most valuable techniques in the area of sensory-motor performance as evidenced by their extensive utilization in motor-skills psychology (Fleischman, 1972; Poulton, 1974; Schmidt, 1975). Tracking tasks have a continuously varying input signal which the subject must attempt to match as closely as possible with his/her output. There are three basic categories of tracking task differing primarily in terms of their visual display and the corresponding control systems. For instance

Figure 5.4 Thompson digital switch.

BBC microcomputer

Thompson digital switch

Quadriceps switch equipment

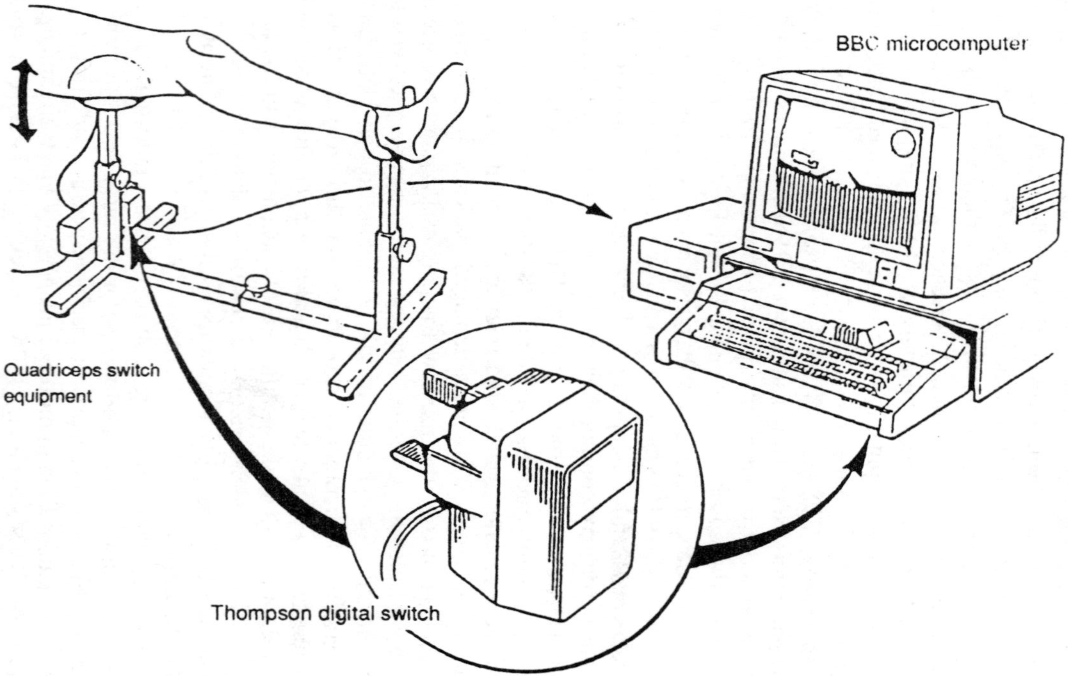

the pursuit task displays both the present input and output signals, whereas the compensatory task displays only the difference or error signal between these displays. The preview task is similar to the pursuit task except that the patient can see in advance where the input signal is to appear and plan accordingly to minimize the resultant error signal. Hence, in a typical paradigm, the patient might manually follow a circuit drawn out.

Performance on a tracking task makes continuous demands on the upper-limb sensory-motor system: visual sensing and perceiving of the display signals in terms of absolute position and velocity, interpretation of this information and the planning of motor actions considered most likely to minimize resultant errors, motor execution requiring smooth co-ordinated arm movements in controlling the output transducer, and integration with somatic sensations from the limb. Continuous-performance feedback through the visual display involves learning processes amenable to investigation. In addition to measurement of integrated function, tracking is suitable for analysis using engineering control theories which can lead to further investigation on underlying neurological control mechanisms (Parker *et al.*, 1979) such as those involved in stroke.

Considering the substantial use made of tracking tasks by psychologists (especially in North America) in investigations of normal motor skills, the application of tracking tasks to the neurologically disabled is surprisingly limited and usually restricted to the conventional pursuit rotor (which is a device for enabling these measurements). Although the pursuit rotor (Ryan, 1962) has a place in the measurement of hand-eye co-ordination, its limitations (periodic input only, inflexible output transducer, extremely crude error detection) make it inferior as a research or clinical tracking type task. Only tracking tasks with an oscilloscope or teletype display are considered in the following review of their use in clinical neurology.

Cassell, Shaw and Stern (1973) used a random input pursuit tracking task with a horizontal movable arm rest to measure the elbow movement of parkinsonian patients on drug trials. Average relative amplitude and average delay errors made by patients were computed from cross-correlation analysis. They demonstrated that the tracking task closely followed varying clinical events in comparison with more conventional tests of motor function such as pegboard, tapping and reaction performances which did not alter significantly. However, the use of pursuit tracking tasks with stroke patients is not well documented.

Flowers (1976) used a variable step pursuit tracking task with a joystick to investigate characteristics of voluntary movement in terms of duration, velocity and accuracy of step responses. He found that certain gross movements were slowed down in parkinsonian patients but not in patients with intention tremor (such as those that had suffered stroke). (Potvin and Tourtellotte (1975) developed a tracking task test battery as a component in a comprehensive clinical quantitative neurological examination. The tracking task was operated in pursuit or compensatory modes with either a position stick, involving primarily shoulder rotation, or a force stick as an output transducer. Although a variety of analyses were performed on the random tracking test data, the most clinically useful measure was found to be the average absolute error. Several other measures derived from cross-correlation analysis were considered to be neither reliable nor valid for parkinsonian or multiple sclerosis patients. The test battery also included a 'critical' task (Jex, McDonnell and Patah, 1986) and a pursuit rotor.

Other clinical applications have included the Lynn et al. (1977) and De Souza et al. (1980) studies. These investigations used a random input pursuit tracking task with a horizontal steering wheel requiring both shoulder and elbow movements. Their work revolves primarily around stroke patients, in contrast to the before-mentioned researchers who have dealt mainly with patients with progressive neurological diseases. They have investigated a wide variety of error analysis techniques and have constructed preliminary recovery curves as tools for prognosis and validation of techniques used in rehabilitation management. Results have proved valuable in helping develop theories of the neurological mechanisms involved in tracking and the underlying defects in hemiplegic patients (Parker et al., 1979).

Tracking tasks have also been used clinically with emphasis on their therapeutic qualities. Driscoll (1975) and Newman and Sproull (1979) both used two-dimensional pursuit tracking for children with learning disabilities. These also have potentially useful qualities for adult stroke patients suffering perceptual dysfunction.

6

Database Techniques and Expert Systems

CHRONIC DISEASE DATABASE SYSTEMS

A database is a collection of stored data organized in such a way that all user-data requirements are satisfied by the database. In general there is only one copy of each item of data although there may be controlled repetition of some data.

Basically a chronic disease database system provides access to previous clinical experience and the means to analyse that experience. The American Rheumatism Association (ARA) has developed a multi-centre medical information system (MIS) where patient data, including stratifying variables (i.e. variables that allow the data to be ordered in some way), descriptions of interventions, and detailed patient course and outcome are entered into the data bank using standard protocols to prospectively follow thousands of patients. The database can be interrogated by participants who may then use the information to complement presently available sources of clinical information. Details of this system have been documented by Fries (1976) and Wiederhold (1976).

Using data from 830 patients discharged from a stroke rehabilitation unit, a stroke database has been compiled at the Burke Rehabilitation Centre. Major factors influencing outcome following stroke were identified (Feigenson, McCarthy and Meese, 1977; Feigenson *et al.*, 1977; Feigenson and Greenberg, 1979) and a statistical analysis subsequently showed the relative importance of each of the factors identified as effecting outcome (Feigenson, 1976). Other studies have identified costs and have suggested methods of cost containment for treating patients during the acute and rehabilitative phases of stroke and commented on the effectiveness of different types of programme in modifying outcome (Feigenson and McCarthy, 1977).

FURTHER READING

The following provide detail to the sections covered in the Chapter:

Feedback induced muscular exercise

Gelman, J., Lakie, M., Walsh, E.G. and Wright, G.W. (1978) Treatment of hemiplegia by feedback induced muscular exercise, *Journal of Physiology*, **285**, 6P–7P.

Joint position biofeedback

Koheil, R. and Mandel, A.R. (1980) Joint position biofeedback facilitation of physical therapy in gait training, *American Journal of Physical Medicine*, **59**, 6, 288–97.
Crofts, F. and Crofts, J. (1988) Biofeedback and the computer, *British Journal of Occupational Therapy*, **51**, 2, 57–9.

Sensor pads

Triptree, V.J. and Harrison, M.A. (1980) The use of sensor pads in the treatment of adult hemiplegia, *Physiotherapy*, **66**, 9, 299.

ARAMIS project

Wiederhold, V. (1976) ARAMIS manual, *Project Report*, Department of Immunology, Stanford University Medical Center, Stanford, California, USA.

The utility of a time-oriented data bank (i.e. based on time since onset of stroke) for chronic diseases has already been demonstrated by Fries and co-workers. They worked with eight institutions contributing data on long-term arthritis (ARAMIS) to develop a system for collecting and storing information. This system performs computer consultations, library searches and can search through its memory banks to compare effectiveness of different types of treatment in matched groups. It also can compare outcome and treatment modalities in the different institutions participating in ARAMIS and search out clusters of particular types of arthritis-related disorders for epidemiological investigation.

Ellenberg (1977) has pointed out some potential dangers of using a database system to make global statements regarding prognosis and efficacy of treatment. It is apparent that: (a) very careful attention to quality of data, selection of cases, and statistical procedures employed is required; and (b) conclusions derived from sampling the data should be confirmed by definitive clinical studies. The potential clinical and research applications of this type of time-oriented approach to a stroke database system have spurred further development of the Burke Stroke Time-Oriented Profile (BUSTOP) model.

MICROCOMPUTER-BASED DATA MANAGEMENT SYSTEMS

The introduction of computers, particularly microcomputers has had an impact on most health care professions in Great Britain and the United States. Microcomputers have had their main influence on methods used in the psychological testing of patients and in the retraining of cognitive deficits. These particular aspects have been reviewed on a number of occasions (Thompson, 1984a; 1987d). For psychological testing and considerations before microcomputer usage see Feigenson (1976), Ellenberg (1977), Thompson (1982, 1983a,b,c; 1984b) and the potential contribution of a microcomputer for handling information which is collected about patients has been an important contribution made by Kapur in 1984.

In the Kapur (1984) study three main applications of a data management package were reviewed: (i) as a means of storing records about individuals; (ii) to help in the preparation of clinical reports; and (iii) to assist in clinical decision-making. Although the

147

latter is an extensive field in its own right, most data management packages can be used indirectly to assist in decision making and this is a particular application which clinical psychologists and occupational therapists are finding useful in everyday clinical work.

In the software package developed by Kapur (1984) information may be stored in character, numerical or data form with a maximum of 40 fields (i.e. sub-categories of data) in a record (category of data for storage purposes) with up to 254 characters (alphabetic letters) in a particular field and up to 1016 characters in a whole record. The first and most important task was to design the structure of the record file. This was critical as the structure of the file would largely determine the range of data-manipulation activities which could later be used with other programs in the package. The converse also holds; it is useful first of all to examine the data-manipulation facilities of the package and this will indicate what constraints, if any, one should consider when designing the structure of a file. The content of each field and the number of fields to be used will vary according to the particular needs of the specific application.

The neuropsychological records used in the study comprised three types of information: biographical data, medical information and psychological test scores. The 'key field' was the patient's name; duplicate keys, while being possible, were discouraged as this results in slower record retrieval when records are accessed on the basis of the key field. Standard biographical information was included in the first few fields. Clinical information was stored in a set of subsequent fields. An important piece of clinical information is that which classifies a patient's condition – this may range from a diagnostic classification to a classification denoting the reason for referral of the patient. A number of medical classification systems already exist but in this study, a purpose-built classification was developed.

Using this system patients could be classified in a number of ways and these included disease aetiology, area of brain involved and type of psychological disorder displayed by the patient. Each of the types of classification was given a unique alphanumeric code such that the patients who had a specific feature who fell into a certain category of features could be subsequently selected. Using codes in this way, instead of a literal description of the patient's features, saves space in the record file. As a general rule, using codes for information in record files will save computer space but this benefit is always to be weighed against the time spent in consulting (and deciphering) the code in question, despite its clear security advantages (with respect to protecting patient confidentiality).

Retrieval facilities are the next important feature from the point of view of clinical use. The features within this package were quite powerful and permitted selection on the basis of particular information in a specified field, part of a field or set of fields. Fields which contained a specified string of characters could also be used for selecting information from patient records.

A final, important feature of a data management package with respect to record filing is the ability to change the structure of a file after a number of records have already been stored. This facility avoids the tedious task of having to create a new file and to key-in all the old records in the new format. The particular package which is now being used by Kapur at the Wessex Neurological Centre in Southampton, England, allows the user such a facility and also enables changes to be made to the names of specific fields.

Conclusions on microcomputer-based data management systems

Preferred features of data management systems for clinical record filing are:

1. Ability to allow for a large number of fields (at least 100);
2. Ability to change file structure easily;
3. Multi-field access (i.e. ability to retrieve information from several different categories of data);
4. Good retrieval facilities including the ability to search parts of a field for pre-defined character strings;
5. Good report generation facilities which incorporate word processing features;
6. Ability to link the data management package with a statistical package.

Preferred hardware features to support such a system include 16–bit architecture and 256K RAM (Random Access Memory) – which are terms used to describe the configuration and memory capacity of the computer – since a number of the better database-packages only function in such environments. Hard-disc storage facilities are useful only if one anticipates accessing more than

149

several hundred patient records at a time and if speed of access is important in the particular working situation.

With regard to security, a data management package should permit data files to be accessed only after entry of a character (numeric or alphanumeric) password. Some packages permit different levels of security controls to be used depending on the amount of information to be made available for inspection. With respect to most of the data on record files, providing that they are in fully-coded formats, if they were viewed by an unauthorized individual, it is doubtful whether the data would be very meaningful.

INTRODUCTION TO EXPERT SYSTEMS

An expert system is a computer system which manifests the capabilities of a human expert in some area of human activity. Expert systems constitute a branch of artificial intelligence, the discipline whose objective is to create machines with some degree of 'intelligence'. A comprehensive definition of expert systems has been approved by the British Computer Society's Committee of its specialist group on expert systems and reads as follows:

An expert system is regarded as the embodiment within a computer of a knowledge-based component from an expert skill in such a form that the system can offer *intelligent advice* or take an *intelligent decision* about a processing function. A desirable additional characteristic, which many would consider fundamental, is the capability of the system, on demand to *justify its own line of reasoning* in a manner directly intelligible to the enquirer. The style adopted to attain these characteristics is *rule-based programming.*

However, this definition leaves much to be desired. For instance, using rules is just one possible way of encoding knowledge, and to infer that this is essential is too categoric. There are many alternative definitions, both broader and narrower than this one and it is often the case that the term expert system is used very loosely and requires additional explanation and details. It is perhaps useful to cite a well known expert system by way of example – the one chosen is MYCIN whose expertise is that of the diagnosis and treatment of infectious diseases.

In operation, MYCIN first collects from the doctor all relevant information about a particular patient and then produces a diagnosis and recommendation for therapy. This process takes place in four stages:

1. Determining if the patient has a significant infection and if so;
2. Determining the likely identity of the offending organism(s);
3. Deciding which drug(s) are likely to be most effective in general, and;
4. Choosing the most effective drug(s) for the patient.

The following can be said of MYCIN:

1. It is rule-based;
2. It establishes information about the specific circumstances for this consultation by asking questions;
3. It reasons about the information presented to it;
4. It can replace its reasonings;
5. It presents conclusions and can also present alternative, less likely conclusions;
6. It uses an inference mechanism which does not associate complete certainty with each fact.

MYCIN is an interactive system (between user and machine) designed to offer expert level medical advice about patients with acute infections. MYCIN's knowledge is stored as fact triples (i.e. if x and y are true then z must be true) with associated degrees of certainty, and as conditional rules relating facts (i.e. z is true if fact x is satisfied).

Attempts are constantly being made to apply expert systems to a wide variety of problems. Different problem areas require expert systems with different characteristics. This leads to the idea of categorizing expert systems according to the functions they perform. For instance, the following have been suggested:

1. Interpretative: the analysis of observable data to which some kind of symbolic meaning may be attached (e.g. in a prognostic expert system for stroke, a set of symptoms may indicate a poor or good prognosis (Thompson, 1987f);
2. Diagnostic: diagnostic systems identify a fault and may prescribe a remedy. Complications may arise when one fault interferes with another, faults are intermittent, or when

complete fault data is not available;

3. Monitor: these systems continuously interpret observable data and compare an interpretation of it with some expectation about the system;

4. Predictive: these forecast the future from a model of the past and present (e.g. the prognosis of a stroke patient). For an expert system to be useful there must be incomplete information so that predictions can be made;

5. Planner: the preparation of a program of actions to be carried out to achieve a set of goals;

6. Designer: in this case the system must create some object (e.g. a circuit, a building, a garment) to meet specification. This is the most open-ended and potentially difficult to implement of all categories.

Before it can be used, the expert system must be built. This is by no means a trivial task. Leaving until later the fundamental questions of knowledge representation and inference, it is still necessary to find a source of expertise for the expert system to impart. One possibility arises in the case of written regulations, rules, laws, etc. These can be analysed and coded directly. More typically the expertise is knowledge known to an expert, but not written down. It may be quite abstruse and technical, but it may be no more than a set of rules-of-thumb known only to a few people, such as that knowledge imparted by occupational therapists during stroke prognosis.

When a human expert has expertise that is to be entered in the expert system, this must be elicited from him or her. Often this is done by a knowledge engineer in a series of discussions with the expert. The process is a surprisingly lengthy one which may take many consultations. Usually a prototype is built and this is interactively improved as each discussion uncovers more expertise or reveals deficiencies in what has already been entered into the expert system.

A simple expert system may eventually reach a state when it is considered to be finished and ready to be put into production without further modification. But for the more complex systems, it seems there is a continual need to update and improve. This may reflect the changing nature of what constitutes expert knowledge in the chosen domain.

In designing an expert system, regard must be made to the type of person who is to use it. It may be that the user will have no technical knowledge at all. This would be true of certain advisory expert systems, e.g. to give advice to claimants about social security benefit. But quite often, as with MYCIN, the user is assumed to have a considerable amount of background knowledge to bring to consultation and to make sense of the system's expertise.

Many different approaches have been taken to expert system construction, and no one model of their organization will adequately represent them all. However, the following constituents are generally accepted, although in practice, the boundaries between these components are often vague:

1. Data: the facts in some particular situation (e.g. the stroke patient has a history of angina pectoris);
2. Knowledge-base: general statements relating particular facts and classes of facts, usually with an implied or explicit conclusion, or action or procedure (e.g. if the stroke patient has a lesion in the right hemisphere, he/she will be left-side-affected);
3. Control (inference mechanism): the mechanism for sequencing through the knowledge-base and activating the statements therein (e.g. if the stroke patient has a cerebral aneurysm, then check data for probability of rupturing and issue appropriate statements).

It is also useful to consider how this knowledge would be stored and accessed:

1. Acquisition: bringing new knowledge into the knowledge-base, and possibly interfering with the performance of knowledge already held in the base (e.g. addition of new stroke patient data);
2. Retrieval: determining what knowledge is relevant to a given problem, a task at which humans are very efficient (e.g. if the stroke patient is over 65 years, is the stroke cerebral thrombosis?);
3. Reasoning: produces new facts and knowledge from existing facts and knowledge (e.g. if x stroke patients who suffer from angina have a poor prognosis, then the probability of stroke patient A, who has angina, having a poor prognosis is y). However, in humans, there seems to be several types of reasoning: formal (using rules of inference and logic);

procedural (using simulation to answer problems); analogical (by analogy); generalization and abstraction; and meta-level reasoning (reasoning about reasoning).

Having established the structural framework of the expert system, the contents (i.e. the information) can then be investigated in further detail. However, it should be noted that the end result (i.e. what information the expert system contains, and how it is to be used) must be kept in mind at all times so that the framework can be adapted according to the needs of the user. For example, on setting out to build an expert system it may be decided that a designer type of system is required, when in reality what may be more appropriate is a predictive expert system, as would be the case with an expert system for stroke prognosis.

ANALYSING DATA STATISTICALLY FOR USE IN EXPERT SYSTEMS

There are a host of statistical tests and computer packages which can be used to assist in the analysis of data for use in a future expert system. Three well-known statistical techniques will be considered here which were used to analyse the data collected in the Thompson and Coleman (1987g) research. For the data collected from the National Stroke Survey, Spearman's Coefficient of Rank Correlation was used to discern any correspondence between variables (i.e. stroke factors) detailed in the survey. For example, to determine if age range was correlated with the particular type of stroke presented. The second technique, the Automatic Interaction Detector (AID) sought a pattern in the variables of the survey: it examined all the data by splitting them into different groups which, within the groups, were related. For instance, all the patients found to have an ischaemic stroke, a poor prognosis and were poorly motivated, may have been placed together, thus providing a percentage for each type of grouping. The third technique, multidimensional scaling (MDS), represented all these stroke factors spatially – their position in relation to poor or good prognosis representing their degree of association, or frequency of occurrence with this prognosis.

Finally, in order to address the problem of uncertainty in any prediction, it was considered essential to have a probability component to the model. Therefore, conditional probability formulae were used to predict the occurrence of each stroke factor used in the survey with a poor or good prognosis. Thus, it was possible to quote probability values, for example, for the probability of a patient with a non-ischaemic stroke having a poor prognosis (based on the sample and as a prediction for the wider unknown stroke population). This final component constituted the actual model of stroke prognosis.

Additional more complex data (EMG data and reaction time scores which had previously been examined statistically using statistical significance tests), were also subjected to these conditional probability formulae so that they too become incorporated into the model. These analytical steps are now described in further detail as an example of how such data can be organized for the construction of an expert system.

The factors of the survey referred to those parameters which the respondents (occupational therapists from around the country) were asked to complete for each patient (i.e. age, sex, type of stroke, etc.). The frequency of occurrence of each of these factors being associated with (a) a poor prognosis; and (b) a good prognosis, was found by summing the occurrences when they were found with a poor and good prognosis for each patient detailed.

Spearman's coefficient of rank correlation

Since it was not known whether data followed the pattern of the normal distribution (i.e. a bell-shaped graph that many data follow), the non-parametric Spearman's Coefficient of Rank Correlation Test was used to identify any factors that were positively or negatively correlated (see Correlation in Glossary). As the sample size of 94 patients exceeded the range of tabulated values for the test, two transformations were necessary: (i) an adjustment to the calculated correlations so they approximated to the t-distribution (another distribution commonly used in statistics); and (ii) an adjustment to the tabulated values of the t-distribution using Z scores (derived from the data using statistical formulae) of the normal distribution. (These will not be discussed further here, but the reader is referred to Thompson, 1987f, where a full explanation may be found).

Since correlation analysis is meaningful only with ordinal data (i.e. data that can be ordered, as compared with nominal data), only pairs of ordinal factors were chosen to determine whether or not a correlation existed between them. Every pair-combination of all the available ordinal factors were tested:

Code letters	Pairs of factors compared
AB	Age range and number of previous strokes
AC	Age range and number of weeks post-stroke
AD	Age range and motivation
AE	Age range and graded symptoms
BC	Number of previous strokes and number of weeks post-stroke
BD	Number of previous strokes and motivation
BE	Number of previous strokes and graded symptoms
CD	Number of weeks post-stroke and motivation
CE	Number of weeks post-stroke and graded symptoms
DE	Motivation and graded symptoms

Correlations were calculated for each pair of factors (over all 94 patients) with the following results:

Pairs of stroke factors	+VE/−VE correlations	Converted t values	% Significance
AB	0.61	7.38	$^1/_2$
AC	−0.99	−67.31	$^1/_2$
AD	−0.76	−11.22	$^1/_2$
AE	0.88	17.77	$^1/_2$
BC	−0.75	−10.88	$^1/_2$
BD	0.01	0.10	not signif
BE	0.70	9.40	$^1/_2$
CD	−1.00	infinity	$^1/_2$
CE	−1.00	infinity	$^1/_2$
DE	−0.72	−9.95	$^1/_2$

This means that in all but one case (i.e. BD, which was the pair 'number of previous strokes and motivation') there were strong correlations found at the $\frac{1}{2}$% level (with $t > 2.63$) of the statistical significance (i.e. $99\frac{1}{2}$ times in 100 chance of finding this evidence). Hence, the following can be said of the data based on these results (see also Figure 6.1):

1. Age range is positively correlated with number of previous strokes;
2. Age range is positively correlated with graded symptoms;
3. Number of previous strokes is positively correlated with graded symptoms;
4. Age range is negatively correlated with number of weeks post-stroke;
5. Age range is negatively correlated with motivation;
6. Number of previous strokes is negatively correlated with number of weeks post-stroke;
7. Number of weeks post-stroke is negatively correlated with motivation;
8. Number of weeks post-stroke is negatively correlated with graded symptoms;

Figure 6.1 Strong positive/negative correlations between stroke factors.

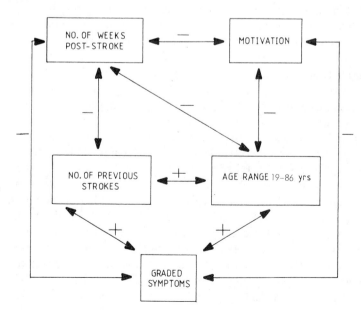

9. Motivation is negatively correlated with graded symptoms;
10. There was no evidence of a correlation between number of previous strokes and motivation.

In summary, the older stroke patients had higher incidences of previous strokes with more high-graded symptoms and tended to be in the group that were recently recovering from the cerebrovascular accident (i.e. only a few weeks post-stroke). This group also had lower motivation. In support of this, correlations were also found between the number of weeks post-stroke and motivation (negatively correlated) and graded symptoms (negatively correlated). However there was no evidence of a correlation between the number of previous strokes and motivation. These factors were then considered in the global context of functional outcome by using a computerized interaction detector.

Automatic interaction detector

Another mathematical option also available is a computerized facility known as the Automatic Interaction Detector (Sonquist, Baker and Morgan, 1973). This was developed by two Americans, John A. Sonquist and James N. Morgan, who were dissatisfied with standard cross-tabulation analyses and their inability to reveal complex interactions in survey data, and follows from the early well-known work of Dr William A. Belson who devised the multivariate matching technique, the Belson Sort. The Automatic Interaction Detector examines data from an input data file (see Glossary definition) and calculates the mean and between sum of squares (see Glossary definition) from each data point (in the case of the survey this was from each frequency of occurrence). Data is read for each category (e.g. stroke factor) and also for each subcategory (e.g. for type of stroke this was ischaemic, non-ischaemic, and unknown CVA). By splitting this data at the point of highest between sum of squares, the data makes a journey along an underlying tree structure (i.e. calculations are made depending on choices at different branches of the route) which identifies the most significant interaction of the data set (of variables). This is best explained by example. The split by the Automatic Interaction Detector of the national stroke survey data may be represented according to the following block diagram (Figure 6.2).

As seen in this diagram, there are cases when the sample size

Figure 6.2 Stroke factor splits using Automatic Interaction Detector.

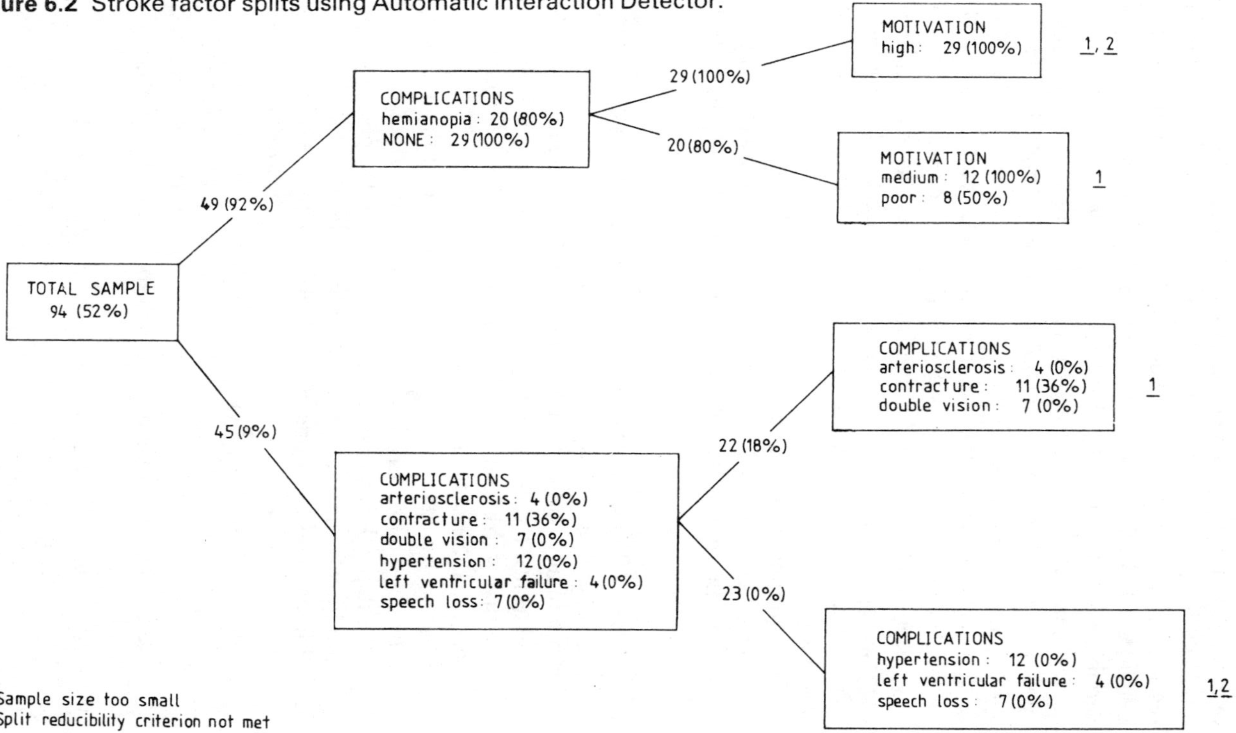

TOTAL SAMPLE
94 (52%)

49 (92%)

45 (9%)

COMPLICATIONS
hemianopia : 20 (80%)
NONE : 29 (100%)

COMPLICATIONS
arteriosclerosis : 4 (0%)
contracture : 11 (36%)
double vision : 7 (0%)
hypertension : 12 (0%)
left ventricular failure : 4 (0%)
speech loss : 7 (0%)

29 (100%)

20 (80%)

22 (18%)

23 (0%)

MOTIVATION
high : 29 (100%)

1, 2

MOTIVATION
medium : 12 (100%)
poor : 8 (50%)

1

COMPLICATIONS
arteriosclerosis : 4 (0%)
contracture : 11 (36%)
double vision : 7 (0%)

1

COMPLICATIONS
hypertension : 12 (0%)
left ventricular failure : 4 (0%)
speech loss : 7 (0%)

1, 2

1 – Sample size too small
2 – Split reducibility criterion not met

159

may be too small for the data to be represented. This is very often the case because the user sets the critical sample size; hence extreme caution is warranted when interpreting results from such an analysis. Similar pitfalls have been detailed by a number of researchers (e.g. Sonquist, Baker and Morgan, 1971; Doyle and Fenwick, 1975). One problem of the technique is that it selects the variable with the highest between sum of squares (BSS) or total sum of squares (TSS) in order to split the sample. All subsequent splits are then contingent on the sub-groups formed by the first split. Yet it is possible a second variable is almost as discriminating as the first. Had the Automatic Interaction Detector program split by this second variable, the subsequent tree data structure might have been totally different. Other 'near misses', as Assael (1970) suggests could markedly change the characters of progressive splits. However, this problem can be partially resolved by judicious use of the program.

The Automatic Interaction Detector may be used for nominal or ordinal data but is limited in its use as are other analytical programs. In short, the following recommendations have been advised:

1. At least 1000 variables should be used if meaningful results are to be obtained. However, this number may be substantially reduced if the Automatic Interaction Detector is used as just a pointer to direct the user to the areas of the data that warrant further explanation or analysis (Sonquist, Baker and Morgan, 1971);
2. Where correlated predictors are present, one of them is likely to be chosen exclusively (Doyle and Fenwick, 1975);
3. If the dependent variable is heavily skewed, the program may tend to split off small groups (Sonquist, 1970);
4. Although early versions of the Automatic Interaction Detector give a significance test for splits, they ignore the basic search strategy followed by the algorithm (set of procedures for making a calculation). Sonquist, Baker and Morgan (1973) admit that: 'because of the large number of possible splits examined there is no point asking about significance';
5. Despite the explicit goal of identifying structure, the Automatic Interaction Detector is found to be insensitive to various forms of interaction. Since it only examines the immediate effect of a predictor on BSS and not future splits,

any interactions which are not 'one-stage' will not be identified (Doyle and Fenwick, 1975).

In summary it can be said of the Automatic Interaction Detector that caution must be made when using the program even when different samples are drawn from the same population, as it is unlikely that an identical tree structure will be obtained (Sonquist, 1970). However, it is a worthwhile first step before applying conditional probability formulae for specific factors, and if each split (or branch in the tree) is noted, the Automatic Interaction Detector can provide a useful indication of the general form of the data presented.

The Automatic Interaction Detector was thus used as a rough guide to discern any underlying pattern in the survey data collected. Using it for the 16 stroke factors used in the survey and with functional outcome (i.e. poor or good prognosis) being the dependent variable, the following results were most salient:

1. Patients with a good prognosis had:
   no complications (64.4%);
   drugs for anticoagulance (69.6%);
   high motivation (70.5%);
2. Patients with a poor prognosis had:
   hypertension (52.2%);
   drugs for hypertension (52.2%);
   poor motivation (100%).

The Automatic Interaction Detector thus highlighted some of the combinations of stroke factors that present with a poor and a good prognosis which were useful at the construction stage of the stochastic model (i.e. a model based on probability). Reference was then given by Thompson (1987f) and Thompson and Coleman (1987f) to these areas during the calculation of conditional probabilities for functional outcome.

Multidimensional scaling (MDS)

Multidimensional scaling (MDS) refers to a family of models by means of which information contained in a set of data is represented by a set of points in a space. These points are arranged in such a way that geometrical relationships such as distance between the points reflect the empirical relationships in the data. For example, the complex associations between a set of variables which are contained in a matrix of correlations can be represented spatially by portraying each variable as a point, placing them in such a way that the distance between them reproduces the numerical value of the correlation coefficients. Thus, a picture of the data is produced which is much easier to assimilate (visually) than a large matrix of numbers. It may well also bring out features of the data which were obscured in the original matrix of coefficients. (The reader is referred to Coxon, (1982) and to Thompson (1987) for fuller explanations about MDS).

The MDS technique thus involves successive iterations on a data configuration, re-fitting data to a new configuration, finding the disparities in fitting the new data, determining the new 'Euclidean' distance (Coxon, 1982), and finally representing them spatially. Since there may be many (i.e. hundreds) of progressive iterations, a computer is best suited to cope with the laborious mathematics involved.

For this reason SPSS–X (2.1) – Statistical Package for the Social Sciences (SPSS, 1986) – was used to perform a statistical analysis of the survey data in the Thompson and Coleman (1987f) study. The raw survey data was used to create a digital file in VIEW (the word processor facility of the Acorn BBC micro-computer series) and then uploaded from floppy disc to become a system file on ICL 2960 mainframe on which a version of SPSS–X (2.1) was installed.

The first stage of analysis was the establishment of a set of proximities (a term used to describe the arrangement of data that has been related in some way) from the survey data. This meant finding a way of representing these discrete interval data (see Glossary definition) in terms of their degree of similarity or dissimilarity to each other. A convenient statistical test that can be used to highlight such a relationship among data is the Chi Squared Test. But since MDS Euclidean Distance matrices by convention show the dissimilarities between variables, a Reverse Chi Squared Test was used instead which meant that each resulting value bore a negative sign. These proximity measures were then presented for MDS analysis where successive iterations were performed comprising the data-fitting and distance calculations previously described.

According to Euclidean Theory, the greater the number of spatial dimensions used to plot a given data set, the 'truer' the representation. Two dimensions can offer data in only two directions in which to be spatially represented (their distance apart reflecting their dissimilarity or in this case their degree of similarity to each other); greater than two dimensions can therefore offer a better spatial fit for the data. In general, the higher the dimensionality of the solution, the easier it is to fit the information, and therefore the lower the 'stress' value (Coxon, 1982).

Since it was of interest to determine which points from the survey data were clustered around (and therefore contributed in some way to) the variable point 'prognosis', rather than the relationship (and spatial distance) between each variable, it was considered sufficient to perform the MDS analysis up to a maximum of four dimensions. In any case, beyond 3-D analysis, it becomes increasingly difficult to (a) represent visually; and (b) 'picture' conceptually. Therefore, the results of MDS were interpreted from two, three and four dimensions only. (The results of one of these interpretations is shown in Figure 6.3).

For technical reasons, the computer begins calculating its solutions in four dimensions. After all, it is easier to fit the data in the greatest possible number of dimensions and then to progressively attempt to find a slightly inferior fit for the data in less dimensions. However, the more dimensions used the less clear is the interpretation and visual representation becomes increasingly difficult! At best, the 4-D solution, for instance, can be represented in a table showing the order of nearness of each of the variables to the point (or variable) of interest.

In summary, the following can be said of these solutions from MDS analysis. As the number of spatial dimensions decreased the order of variables appears to change; probably the most noticeable in position during derivation of stimulus configurations was AFFECT (affected side) in the 4–D solution. But the variable TYPE (type of strokes) was also of interest in being particularly consistently placed (in order of nearness to PROGNOSIS). Therefore, the following variables were identified as having possible importance to the functional outcome (i.e. PROGNOSIS) of a stroke (not in order of importance since this cannot be discerned solely by MDS analysis and when 'weighting' was not possible to implement):

- Affect (affected side);
- Complic (medical complications);
- Condit (medical conditions);

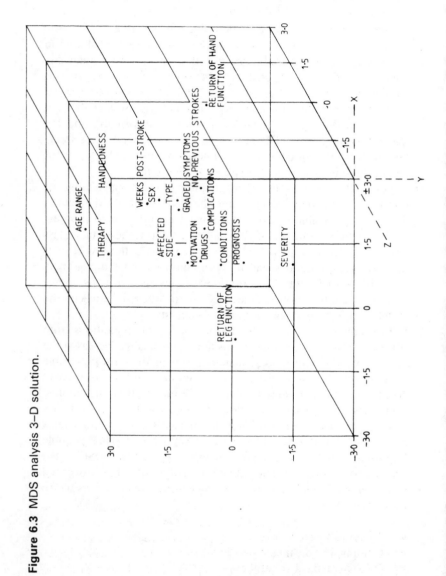

Figure 6.3 MDS analysis 3–D solution.

- Drugs (administered);
- Gradsym (graded neurological symptoms);
- Motive (motivation);
- Sever (severity of stroke);
- Sex (of patient);
- Therapy (undertaken);
- Type (type of stroke).

Relative merits of the analytical techniques

Spearman's Coefficient of Rank Correlation Test is a useful technique to use on the survey data since it identifies combinations of stroke factors that occur. For example, it is useful to know that as the number of weeks post-stroke increased (i.e. the greater the time period after the stroke) the motivation of the patient decreased. Thus, the occupational therapist needs to be aware of this during the rehabilitation of the patient so that every effort is made to maintain motivation during the weeks following the CVA. However, this technique can also be used dangerously if it is not remembered that a correlation between two factors does not necessarily imply a causal correlation (see Glossary definition).

Similarly, the automatic interaction detector should also be used with some caution. It was extremely useful in providing an overall rough picture of the data and indicated the percentage of patients falling into particular categories. For instance, 41 patients at the first split of data had a poor prognosis of which four suffered from arteriosclerosis. As this technique has been the subject of much controversy over the years it was decided that these results would be considered cautiously; thus, it was the use of the multi-dimensional scaling (MDS) technique that helped to further confirm or highlight the results of this analysis.

This latter technique was particularly useful in that it overcame the problems faced by many other statistical approaches in not being able to provide a visual picture of the analysis. MDS indicates the spatial relationships of the stroke factors which, in the case of the survey data, helped to identify those factors which the other two techniques had previously picked out. Therefore, the combination of these three techniques was important rather than a reliance on any one, and as is often the case; the results of all three techniques were carefully considered, with heedance to their limitations, so that the conditional probability of occurrence could be calculated for a list of stroke factors which were investigated further with a new sample of stroke patients.

FURTHER READING

Use of computers for patient prognosis

Smith, A.H. (1978) The assessment of patient prognosis using an interactive computer program, *International Journal of Biomedical Computing*, **9**, 1, 37–44.

Expert systems

Although these texts are not specifically related to stroke, the first is a good introduction to the subject; the second is rather esoteric but nonetheless a useful reference text.

Sell, P.S. (1985) *Expert Systems – A Practical Introduction*, Macmillan, Basingstoke.

Waterman, D.A. (1986) *A Guide to Expert Systems*, Addison-Wesley, Reading.

Acquisition of knowledge for a stroke prognosis model

Thompson, S.B.N. (1987) A stochastic model of cerebrovascular accident prognosis, *PhD Thesis*, School of Information Science, Portsmouth Polytechnic, Portsmouth.

Thompson, S.B.N. and Coleman, M.J. (1987) Stroke recovery model, *Therapy Weekly*, **14**, 9, 7.

Automatic interaction detector and multi-dimensional scaling

Coxon, A.P.M. (1982) *The User's Guide to Multidimensional Scaling*, Heinemann, London.

Sonquist, J.A., Baker, E.L. and Morgan, J.N. (1973) *Searching for Structure: An Approach to Substantial Bodies of Micro-Data and Documentation for a Computer Program*, Institute for Social Research, Ann Arbor, Michigan.

Spearman's Coefficient of Rank Correlation may be found in most good non-parametric texts.

7

Expert Systems for Stroke in Occupational Therapy

A MODEL OF STROKE PROGNOSIS

Computer-assisted medical decision-making is becoming better known (Reggia, 1982) with technology advancing so quickly that even the legalities of using such systems are being examined (Arthur, 1986). However, all these systems must have rules and these rules are based on a theory or on extensive knowledge acquired in the field of the expert.

As Spiegelhalter and Knill-Jones (1984) have suggested, where uncertainty exists in these fields, such as in science or in medicine, it should be reliably quantified using appropriate statistical methods, e.g. Bayesian Inference and Decision (Winkler, 1972). Such techniques have been used for predicting the aetiology of stroke (Zagoria and Reggia, 1983), with conclusions that cite strong support for the transferability of Bayesian classification systems to new sites in medicine, e.g. medical decision making in neurology (Salamon, Bernadet and Samson, 1976). Furthermore, this particular study provided support for the utility of clinical databases in building, transferring, and testing Bayesian classification systems in general.

In the application of stroke prognosis it is useful to complete the relationship among identified factors thought to contribute to a good prognosis. A convenient formula that gives relationships among variables is Bayes' Theorem (Winkler, 1972) and named after an English clergyman who conducted early work into probability theory. This theorem can be stated as follows for the probable occurrence of event A given the occurrence of event B, i.e. $p(A|B)$:

$$p(A|B) = \frac{p(B|B) \cdot p(A)}{p(B|A) \cdot p(A) + p(B|A) \cdot p(A)}$$

Where A represents the complement of the event A (that is, 'not A'), and $p(B|A) \cdot p(A)$ means the probability of B given A, multiplied by the probability (i.e. probable occurrence) of A, etc. Sometimes the independence of two events A and B is conditional upon the third event C as follows:

$$p(A, B|C) = p(A|C) \cdot p(B|C)$$

Hence, to find $p(A|C)$ and $p(B|C)$, Bayes' Theorem is used. However, this assumes that each variable is independent of one another (but related to the third event, C). Unless additional information is available concerning this relationship amongst the data, an alternative set of formulae must be used which in fact were involved in the derivation of Bayes' Theorem. Since this is the case with the stroke factors involved in the Thompson and Coleman (1987f) study where each factor may have been related to another, the following conditional probability formulae were used (the example is for a male patient with a severe ischaemic stroke given a poor prognosis):

$$p(\text{ischaemic-stroke} \mid \text{poor-prognosis})$$

$$= \frac{p(\text{ischaemic-stroke, poor-prognosis})}{p(\text{poor-prognosis})}$$

$$= \frac{p(\text{poor-prognosis} \mid \text{ischaemic-stroke}) \cdot p(\text{ischaemic-stroke})}{p(\text{poor-prognosis})}$$

and

$$p(\text{severe-stroke} \mid \text{ischaemic, poor-prognosis})$$

$$= \frac{p(\text{severe, ischaemic, poor})}{p(\text{ischaemic, poor})}$$

$$= \frac{p(\text{ischaemic} \mid \text{severe, poor}) \cdot p(\text{poor} \mid \text{severe}) \cdot p(\text{severe})}{p(\text{ischaemic} \mid \text{poor}) \cdot p(\text{poor})}$$

and

p(male ∣ ischaemic, poor, severe)

$$= \frac{p(\text{male, ischaemic, poor, severe})}{p(\text{ischaemic, poor, severe})}$$

$$= \frac{p(\text{ischaemic} \mid \text{male, poor, severe}).p(\text{poor} \mid \text{male, severe}).\ p(\text{severe} \mid \text{male}).p(\text{severe})}{p(\text{ischaemic, poor, severe})}$$

Where p(male ∣ ischaemic, poor, severe), for example, means the probability of the patient being a male patient given the information that the patient has a severe ischaemic stroke and a poor prognosis; and p(severe, ischaemic, poor) means the probability of these variables occurring together: severe stroke, ischaemic stroke, poor prognosis for the patient, etc.

The probability (of occurrence with a good or poor prognosis) of each variable identified was calculated from the frequency of occurrence in the raw data of the study and from using the conditional probability formulae described. For example, to find the probability of occurrence of an ischaemic stroke with a poor prognosis, the frequency of this presentation (which is f=7/45 from Table 7.1) was entered into the conditional probability formulae as follows:

$$p(A|B) = \frac{p(A,B)}{p(B)} = \frac{p(B|A).p(A)}{p(B)}$$

thus $p(A,B) = p(B|A).p(A)$

so

Table 7.1
Frequency of occurrence for type of stroke (from Thompson, 1987f)

Type of stroke	Poor prognosis	Good prognosis	
ischaemic	7	18	
non-ischaemic	10	6	
unknown CVA	28	25	
TOTAL	45	49	94

169

p(ischaemic-stroke, poor-prognosis) = p(poor-prognosis |
ischaemic-stroke).p(ischaemic-stroke)

$$= \frac{7}{(7+18)} \cdot \frac{(7+18)}{94}$$

$$= 0.07$$

Hence, p = 0.07 for a patient with an ischaemic stroke and a poor
prognosis.

However, if one of these variables is known to be present (just
as with a sample patient being checked using an expert system,
where certain variables or stroke factors are known to be present)
then the probability of, for example, the patient having a poor
prognosis knowing that he/she has an ischaemic stroke is as
follows:

p(B | A) = p(poor-prognosis) | ischaemic-stroke)

$$= \frac{7}{7+18}$$

$$= 0.28$$

It should be noted, however, that p = 0.28 only holds true for
the sample of patients (n = 94) but is an accurate real probability
for this patient-sample based on frequencies. The first probability,
p = 0.07, can only be an estimation for the wider population of
stroke patients since it is calculated from an observation (i.e.
frequencies) from a sample. Hence, p = 0.07 is an estimated
probability. In fact, it is never possible to obtain the exact probability because of the continually changing population due to death,
and of course births of new generations. Hence, for the known
sample of patients, the frequency of occurrence for each variable
(or stroke factor) is the most representative value for that set of
data; but as a predictor or estimator for the larger (unknown)
population of patients falling into good or poor prognosis categories, the estimated probabilities are likely to be more representative. These two values will become closer to each other as more
data is collected, i.e. more information collected for the sample of
patients will make the sample more representative of the (larger)
population of stroke victims. (Probabilities for each variable
identified by the statistical analysis have been included in Tables 7.2
and 7.3).

Table 7.2
Probabilities (and estimated probabilities in parentheses) of
identified stroke factors (from Thompson, 1987f).

Variable(s)	Subcategory(ies)	Poor prognosis	Good prognosis
Affected side	left	0.19 (0.14)	0.81 (0.18)
	right	0.56 (0.44)	0.44 (0.34)
Complications	arteriosclerosis	1.00 (0.04)	0.00 (0.00)
	contracture	0.64 (0.07)	0.36 (0.04)
	double vision	1.00 (0.07)	0.00 (0.00)
	hemianopia	0.20 (0.04)	0.80 (0.17)
	hypertension	1.00 (0.13)	0.00 (0.00)
	left ventricular failure	1.00 (0.04)	0.00 (0.00)
	speech loss	1.00 (0.07)	0.00 (0.00)
	NONE	0.00 (0.00)	1.00 (0.31)
Conditions	angina	0.62 (0.16)	0.37 (0.10)
	diabetes	0.50 (0.05)	0.50 (0.05)
	epilepsy	1.00 (0.05)	0.00 (0.00)
	NONE	0.36 (0.21)	0.64 (0.37)
Drugs for	angina	0.78 (0.07)	0.22 (0.02)
	anticoagulance	0.27 (0.06)	0.73 (0.17)
	arrhythmia	0.45 (0.05)	0.55 (0.06)
	hypertension	0.56 (0.11)	0.44 (0.09)
	muscle spasm	0.45 (0.05)	0.55 (0.06)
	supraventricular arrhythmia	0.80 (0.04)	0.20 (0.01)
	NONE	0.44 (0.09)	0.56 (0.11)
Motivation	high	0.06 (0.02)	0.94 (0.33)
	medium	0.00 (0.00)	1.00 (0.14)
	poor	0.90 (0.46)	0.10 (0.05)

According to Hyland (1981), if the form of an established theory is adopted as the form for a new theory then the established theory is acting as a model for the new. Existing theories based on probabilities about the likelihood of particular medical events can also be used in this way to develop new links between variables through the formulation of modelled theories. For instance, it is

Table 7.3
Probabilities (and estimated probabilities in parentheses) of
identified stroke factors (from Thompson, 1987f).
Continued

Variable(s)	Subcategory(ies)	Poor prognosis	Good prognosis
Severity	mild	0.36 (0.21)	0.64 (0.37)
	severe	0.64 (0.27)	0.36 (0.15)
Type	ischaemic	0.28 (0.07)	0.72 (0.19)
	non-ischaemic	0.62 (0.11)	0.37 (0.06)
	unknown CVA	0.53 (0.30)	0.47 (0.27)
Complications with motivation	arteriosclerosis + high	1.00 (0.01)	0.00 (0.00)
	arteriosclerosis + poor	1.00 (0.03)	0.00 (0.00)
	NONE + high	0.00 (0.00)	1.00 (0.20)
	NONE + medium	0.00 (0.00)	1.00 (0.09)
	NONE + poor	0.00 (0.00)	1.00 (0.02)
Motivation with drugs	high + anticoagulance	0.00 (0.00)	1.00 (0.13)
	high + arrhythmia	0.00 (0.00)	1.00 (0.02)
	high + hypertension	0.00 (0.00)	1.00 (0.05)
	high + muscle spasm	0.33 (0.01)	0.67 (0.02)
	high + NONE	0.09 (0.01)	0.91 (0.11)
	medium + angina	0.00 (0.00)	1.00 (0.02)
	medium + anticoagulance	0.00 (0.00)	1.00 (0.03)
	medium + arrhythmia	0.00 (0.00)	1.00 (0.01)
	medium + hypertension	0.00 (0.00)	1.00 (0.02)
	medium + muscle spasm	0.00 (0.00)	1.00 (0.01)
	poor + angina	1.00 (0.07)	0.00 (0.00)
	poor + anticoagulance	1.00 (0.06)	0.00 (0.00)
	poor + arrhythmia	0.83 (0.05)	0.17 (0.01)
	poor + hypertension	0.83 (0.11)	0.17 (0.02)
	poor + muscle spasm	0.67 (0.04)	0.33 (0.02)
	poor + supraventricular arrhythmia	1.00 (0.04)	0.00 (0.00)
	poor + NONE	1.00 (0.07)	0.00 (0.00)

already known that the survival rate of patients with CVA is not high, with the following estimated probabilities based on a sample of 191 CVA patients (Shafer *et al.*, 1975):

p(surviving 2 days)   = 0.43*
p(surviving 1 month) = 0.23*
p(surviving 1 year)   = 0.15*
p(surviving 3 years) = 0.10*

(*estimated probabilities have been calculated by the authors from Shafer *et al.*, 1975 original frequencies.)

It is also known that out of patients over 65 years old suffering from an initially unknown type of CVA, 90% presented with cerebral thrombosis (Shafer *et al.*, 1975); and that, according to the same source, a cerebral aneurysm commonly ruptures in patients aged 20 years and 40 years with signs and symptoms that can include: sudden explosive headache, photophobia, neck rigidity, nausea and vomiting, loss of consciousness, shock, convulsions, a full bounding pulse and a noisy laboured respiration. Different sources have revealed arteriosclerosis, and hypertension alone (associated with a stroke) as representing some 16% of deaths (Ullman, 1964). These data have already been used to develop theories about the effects of a cerebrovascular accident on victims, including a model that forecasts the recovery of such victims from factors known to be present in patients, e.g. affected side of stroke, reaction time of affected muscle, electrical activity of the incompletely innervated leg, etc. (Thompson, 1987f). Such a model is invaluable to occupational therapists during treatment planning.

From the Thompson and Coleman (1987f) study, electrical activity detected at the quadriceps tendon of tested stroke patients increased with return of function in the lower limbs. These findings were also paralleled by patient's high motivation, but were dependent upon the following pre-requisites: the severity of the stroke was mild; few drugs were administered for few conditions; patients had few or no complications, and the type of stroke was ischaemic.

There was a high probability for these variables occurring with a good prognosis; the confidence levels for the EMG data collected were also reliable (1% and 2.5%), which meant that the probability of obtaining these results under similar conditions by chance were one time in 100 and two and a half times in 100, respectively; clearly very significant results. However, it was important to see how well these findings held for an additional sample of stroke patients, and whether or not they were reliable predictors of a poor or good prognosis. These conclusions were therefore evaluated using a new patient sample, and the results obtained were used to modify the understanding of stroke recovery, and for refinement of the model for incorporation into a prognostic expert system framework. Thus, it has been shown that a series of factors thought to contribute to the recovery of a stroke may be used collectively as a probability model to predict the prognosis of patients whose outcome is unknown.

TESTING A PROGNOSTIC MODEL

To evaluate any proposed model it is best to use a large sample of patients so that any individual differences can hopefully be reduced. However, it is also sometimes difficult to obtain the cross-section and large numbers that would be satisfactory for such an exercise; as with stroke patients, it is time-consuming for both the researcher and therapist to painstakingly collect vast amounts of information which may not always be absolutely necessary. For the Thompson and Coleman (1987g) study, it was only possible to gain access to a suitable cross-section of male outpatients who were attending the outpatient department for occupational therapy. All patients were seen in the department for evaluation and were selected using the criteria of age and number of weeks post-stroke (i.e. were at similar stages of stroke recovery to those patients who had been tested in the earlier study).

The procedure for collecting the EMG data (i.e. the electrical activity from their muscles) from these patients, in addition to testing their quadriceps reactions, was consistent with that adopted for the previous stroke sample of the study. Medical histories were also compiled for each patient and prognoses collected from occupational therapists at this time were checked against the model in order to predict the recovery for the next testing session – hence, this was checked against the actual recovery for each patient four weeks later. In this way, the predictions made by the model could be evaluated and subsequently modified if necessary (Table 7.4).

Patients 01, 02 and 05 were all predicted as having a good prognosis. (It will be noted that where probability values of 1.00 are quoted, additional probabilities are also shown since there is some difference of opinion among statisticians as to the realiability of quoting such values. Therefore, if the reader subscribes to this school of thought, he/she may refer to the next highest probability which is also quoted and which, in all cases, agrees with the first mentioned prediction, i.e. a poor or a good prognosis).

Patients 01, 02 and 05 all showed signs of improved EMG scores, and, as predicted by the stroke factor probabilities, patient 04 showed deterioration as indicated by the muscular reaction time scores. However, there was some inconsistency between this prediction and (a) patient 04's EMG score; and (b) 05's reaction time scores.

Although the results were very encouraging, at this stage it would be unwise to suggest that the model is totally reliable. Clearly, it is not. However, with certain modifications, and with further evaluation, it represents a framework that is then suitable for implementation on a computer system. Some proposals for making these modifications will now be considered.

Proposals for modifying the prognostic model

As with any expert-system model the process of modification and validation is ongoing. Once the initial predictions, made from the earlier study, have been made and evaluated, the model must 'learn' from both its successes and from its failures. As it is a first stage to developing a framework that can be implemented on a computer system, it should be rigorously tested beforehand with a larger number of stroke patients, and cross-validated with experts (occupational therapists and consultants) in the field of stroke rehabilitation. Some suggestions for modifying the model will now be considered:

1. Further testing should be made on a weekly basis, of the EMG and reaction-time scores to discern some pattern, over a large number of patients, that is consistent with the stroke factor predictions;
2. A larger stroke survey should be conducted paying particular notice to those stroke factors with a probability of 1.00 and 0.00. It would be more desirable if these values were slightly less than one and greater than zero, respectively. Such categorical statements, as these values imply, are unlikely, and can be modified as more information is known;

Table 7.4
Comparison between model's predictions and therapists' evaluation of patients at week five (example modified from Thompson, 1987f)

Outpatients	Model's predictions at week one*	Therapists' evaluation at week five
01	p(good-prog. no complications) = 1.00 (0.31) p(good-prog. no conditions) = 0.64 (0.37) p(good-prog. mild stroke) = 0.64 (0.37) p(poor-prog. rt-side-affected) = 0.56 (0.44)	Noticeable improvement in tasks and in walking without assistance
02	p(good-prog. medium-motivation) = 1.00 (0.14) p(poor-prog. hypertension) = 1.00 (0.13) p(good-prog. left-side-affected) = 0.81 (0.18)	Good improvement from week one; now walks unaided although foot drags as before; hand function remains same as before
03	Discharged	Discharged
04	p(poor-prog. speech-loss) = 1.00 (0.07) p(poor-prog. epilepsy) = 1.00 (0.05) p(good-prog. high-motivation) = 0.94 (0.33) p(poor-prog. unknown-CVA) = 0.53 (0.30) p(mild-stroke. good-prog) = 0.37	No noticeable improvement from week one; motivation is reduced; assisted walking with stick; aphasic

05	p(good-prog. high-motivation)	= 0.94 (0.33)	Good return of
	p(poor-prog. non-ischaemic-stroke)	= 0.62 (0.11)	function generally;
	p(rt-side affected. poor-prog)	= 0.44	highly motivated;
	p(no-conditions. good-prog)	= 0.37	walking is good; manual
	p(mild-stroke. good-prog)	= 0.37	dexterity unaffected

*Based on Model's predictions using patients' medical details only (estimated on probabilities in parentheses).

3. By collecting more data the estimated probabilities will tend to approach the values of the observed probabilities (or vice versa), thus making the predictions more accurate;

4. Statistical tests (as used previously) should be used to continually check the significance of data when it is known, thus updating the information contained in the model;

5. The therapists' evaluations should also be statistically correlated with the model's predictions as a check of the reliability of the system. After all, it is the therapist that is ultimately to be emulated (and ideally, with the elimination of human bias!).

CONSTRUCTION OF AN EXPERT SYSTEM FOR STROKE PROGNOSIS

On examination of the findings from the trials detailed in the previous section, the following stroke factors were most salient in predicting the prognosis of the patients tested: complications, motivation of patient, type of stroke, and affected side. Of course, it would be unwise at this stage to rely solely on these factors to predict prognosis of further patients unless a large enough patient sample indicated that this was a valid move to make; however, if such an indication is given, and once the proposed modifications have been completed on the model, the search for a suitable hardware configuration can begin. It would indeed be feasible to use such a system as the Acorn BBC Master Series Micro-computers or even the more advanced Archimedes range to support an expert system for this application. Depending on the size of the final knowledge base, it may in fact be more practical to consider the greater processing and memory capabilities of a personal computer or even a mainframe that could conceivably be accessed by several hospital departments on a network.

This can only be speculative at this stage, but some ideas of what could be expected from such an expert system, based on the tested model, could look like that depicted in Figure 7.1. This shows one of the stroke factors which appears in the model: type of stroke (ischaemic/non-ischaemic/(VA); the system would ask the user to input information about the patient for each of these stroke factors. Depending on the respondent's replies, the system could then navigate the user around a set of subdivisions of the knowledge base (Figures 7.1–7.3), and finally could provide, as

Figure 7.1 Subdivisions of structure of proposed expert system. (From Thompson, 1987f.)

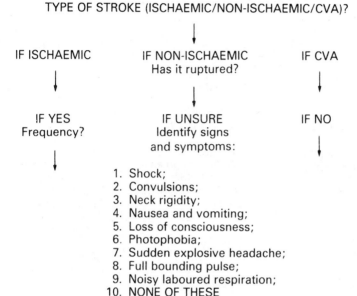

TYPE OF STROKE (ISCHAEMIC/NON-ISCHAEMIC/CVA)?

| IF ISCHAEMIC | IF NON-ISCHAEMIC
Has it ruptured? | IF CVA |

| IF YES
Frequency? | IF UNSURE
Identify signs
and symptoms: | IF NO |

1. Shock;
2. Convulsions;
3. Neck rigidity;
4. Nausea and vomiting;
5. Loss of consciousness;
6. Photophobia;
7. Sudden explosive headache;
8. Full bounding pulse;
9. Noisy laboured respiration;
10. NONE OF THESE

with well-tested systems such as MYCIN and perhaps the less well-known PRECEPTOR (Sell, 1985), a set of explanations to make the system's interactions with the user less ambiguous and thus the respondent's replies (inputs) more accurate. This style of dialogue has been shown to be very successful and in this application could provide a user friendly system such as that depicted in Figure 7.4, which seeks to determine the exact nature of the stroke, (type), which is known to be of importance for the functional outcome and has been addressed by the model. By using a menu-driven program with clear displays for the user's reference, a comprehensive system would then be available for the therapist (Figure 7.5 for an example of a possible screen display).

The development of an expert system for stroke prognosis is by no means a small undertaking. Because of the importance of its recommendations, each stage of the system should be tested and checked by comparison with the equivalent performance of the

Figure 7.2 Subdivisions of structure of proposed expert system (continued) (from Thompson, 1987f).

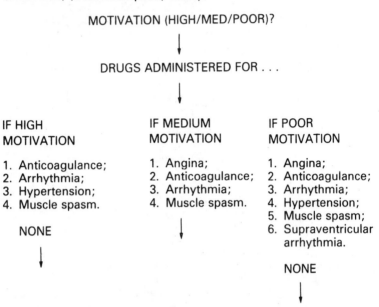

MOTIVATION (HIGH/MED/POOR)?

↓

DRUGS ADMINISTERED FOR . . .

↓

IF HIGH
MOTIVATION

1. Anticoagulance;
2. Arrhythmia;
3. Hypertension;
4. Muscle spasm.

NONE

↓

IF MEDIUM
MOTIVATION

1. Angina;
2. Anticoagulance;
3. Arrhythmia;
4. Muscle spasm.

↓

IF POOR
MOTIVATION

1. Angina;
2. Anticoagulance;
3. Arrhythmia;
4. Hypertension;
5. Muscle spasm;
6. Supraventricular arrhythmia.

NONE

↓

occupational therapist. As with any system that makes predictions when there is uncertainty concerning an outcome of an event or condition, the knowledge base that supports the system is wholly compiled from a large sample – in this case, from a stroke population that is as large as is available and as diverse as possible so that the system's information is representative of the real world. Clearly this may take many years to compile but is nonetheless a fruitful pursuit.

It is expected that such an expert system would be one which fell into one of the categories of expert systems introduced earlier – interpretative (since it would analyse the data that was input and then assign it to a category according to a set of rules) and predictive (since it must forecast the prognosis of the patient from known data). It is likely to be rule-based with an underlining tree structure along which the users are led accordingly to their responses which take them across a variety of branches. This leads on to the next issue which concerns the validity of the system.

As Sell (1985) suggested, the answers given by an expert system should not vary according to extraneous circumstances. This refers

Figure 7.3 Subdivisions of structure of proposed expert system (continued) (from Thompson, 1987f).

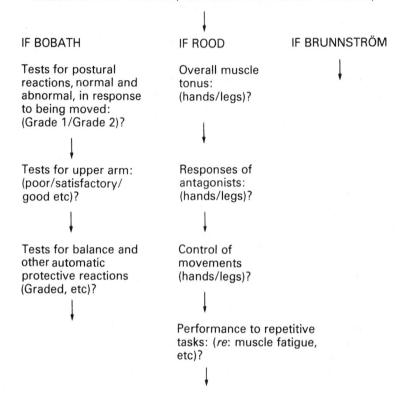

THERAPEUTIC APPROACH (BOBATH/ROOD/BRUNNSTRÖM etc.)?

IF BOBATH

Tests for postural reactions, normal and abnormal, in response to being moved: (Grade 1/Grade 2)?

Tests for upper arm: (poor/satisfactory/good etc)?

Tests for balance and other automatic protective reactions (Graded, etc)?

IF ROOD

Overall muscle tonus: (hands/legs)?

Responses of antagonists: (hands/legs)?

Control of movements (hands/legs)?

Performance to repetitive tasks: (*re*: muscle fatigue, etc)?

IF BRUNNSTRÖM

to the consistency of the system and in this application should be inferred as the unerring ability of the system to make a prognosis without being affected by such variables as the time of day that the system was used or how tired the occupational therapist is who is using the system! Likewise, in order to be consistent the expert system must continually work through the knowledge-base matching the known data with the respondent's inputs in order to make a complete check on the information so that the correct routes are navigated through the system. This idea of completeness is ideological in that any such expert system can only perform such perfect acts in the presence of all known information on the topic, which in turn makes using the expert system redundant since all information is already known. Therefore, one of the limitations of

Figure 7.4 Example dialogue for proposed expert system for stroke prognosis (adapted from Thompson, 1978f).

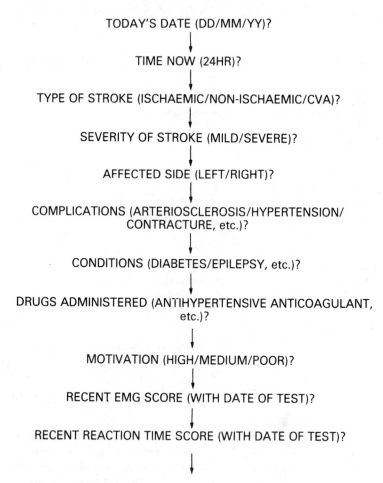

TODAY'S DATE (DD/MM/YY)?

TIME NOW (24HR)?

TYPE OF STROKE (ISCHAEMIC/NON-ISCHAEMIC/CVA)?

SEVERITY OF STROKE (MILD/SEVERE)?

AFFECTED SIDE (LEFT/RIGHT)?

COMPLICATIONS (ARTERIOSCLEROSIS/HYPERTENSION/
CONTRACTURE, etc.)?

CONDITIONS (DIABETES/EPILEPSY, etc.)?

DRUGS ADMINISTERED (ANTIHYPERTENSIVE ANTICOAGULANT,
etc.)?

MOTIVATION (HIGH/MEDIUM/POOR)?

RECENT EMG SCORE (WITH DATE OF TEST)?

RECENT REACTION TIME SCORE (WITH DATE OF TEST)?

the expert system is the extent of the knowledge base from which it consults.

The soundness of the expert system and the precision of the expert system depend largely on how thoroughly comparisons are made with therapists performing similar prognoses. If the expert system produces the same prognosis as a known expert (therapist) then the expert system is sound; if the level of statistical significance of the prognosis given by the expert system is equivalent to that given by the therapist under the same conditions and for the

Figure 7.5 An example of explanations issued for the proposed expert system (from Thompson, 1987f).

Example 1   TYPE OF STROKE?
Why?
Explanation   It is known that of patients over 65 years old presented with an initially unknown CVA, 90% presented with cerebral thrombosis (Shafer *et al.*, 1975).

Example 2   IF STROKE IS NON-ISCHAEMIC, HAS ANEURYSM RUPTURED?
Why?
Explanation   It is known that the probability of survival following a ruptured aneurysm is 50% and that subsequent ruptures reduce prospects of a good prognosis (Shafer *et al.*, 1975).

More Explanation?
Yes?
Explanation   Prospects of a good prognosis following a ruptured aneurysm are further reduced as the age of the patient approaches 40 years — most commonly, rupture occurs in patients aged 20–40 years. Arteriosclerosis and hypertension alone (associated with a stroke) have been found to be responsible for some 16% of deaths (Ullman, 1964).

same patient (knowing the same pool of knowledge) then the expert system is precise.

The issue of useability of expert systems should be discussed. This is very much dependent on the computer language in which the expert system is constructed; how well the user can understand the dialogue; how easy the hardware is to use; and the accessibility of the expert system to the therapist. Other considerations are inevitably the cost of such a system and how quickly the system works – whether or not it can also save the expert's time as well as being equally accurate or even better than the expert under a given set of circumstances.

Finally, it is hoped that such research will indeed be taken a stage further, which should be in the direction discussed in this chapter. Such an expert system would in fact be a highly desirable tool for the occupational therapist bringing the profession up-to-date with the advancements in information technology. As the area of stroke rehabilitation in occupational therapy has so far been a highly subjective and unscientific process, it is believed that such contributions as the computerized assessment batteries (Thompson, 1987b) and stochastic models of stroke prognosis (Thompson, 1987f) return some scientific credibility to the profession, at least in terms of research. However, it is the benefit of stroke patients themselves that this type of research should be about, and it is a measure of success that such programs are beginning to be used in occupational therapy departments in Great Britain and the United States. However, the ultimate measure of success has to be the implementation and use of a prognostic expert system for stroke patients. One hopes that these patients will not have to wait too long!

FURTHER READING

Implications of medical expert systems

Arthur, C. (1986) Who pays if you dial D for diagnosis but end up with death?, *Computer Weekly*, **10**, 1, 28.

Bayesian classification systems: predicting the aetiology of stroke

Zagoria, R.J. and Reggia, J.A. (1983) Transferability of medical decision support systems based on Bayesian classification, *Medical Decision Making*, **3**, 4, 501–9.

Introduction to Bayesian theory

Winkler, R.L. (1972) *An Introduction to Bayesian Inference and Decision*, Holt, Rinehart and Winston, New York.

Glossary

Abduction Drawing of a limb away from midline of body.

Action potential Potential across membrane of active neurone, that is, one that is conducting an impulse. Synonym commonly used for action potential is nerve impulse.

Adduction Drawing of a limb towards midline of body.

Aetiology Cause of disease.

Afferent Designating nerves or neurones that convey impulses to the brain or spinal cord (e.g. Ia and II afferents).

Agnosia Disorder of the brain whereby the patient cannot interpret sensations correctly although the sense organs and nerves conducting sensation to the brain are functioning normally.

Alzheimer's disease Progressive form of dementia occuring in middle age, for which there is no treatment. Associated with diffuse degeneration of the brain.

Aneurysm Balloon-like swelling in wall of an artery, due to disease or congenital deficiency.

Antagonists Muscles that normally produce opposite movement to that of prime movers. They reciprocate with prime movers by adapting in length.

Aphasia Disorder of language affecting generation of speech and its understanding. Caused by disease in left half of brain (the dominant hemisphere) in a right-handed person.

Apraxia Inability to make skilled movements with accuracy. Disorder of cerebral cortex most often caused by disease of the parietal lobes of the brain.

Arthrodial A kind of articulation where the surfaces are either plane, or convex and concave respectively.

Associated reactions Contractions of muscle groups throughout the whole body musculature that accompany voluntary movements especially those performed with effort. In the normal person they increase muscle tone in normal patterns. In the patient with Central Nervous System disorder associated reactions increase muscle tone in abnormal or spastic patterns.

Autonomic nervous system The part of the nervous system responsible for the control of bodily functions that are not consciously directed, including regular beating of the heart, intestinal movements, sweating, salivation, etc.

Axon Nerve-cell-process that transmits impulses away from cell body.

Babinski reflex Upward movement of the great toe that is an abnormal plantar reflex indicating disease in brain or spinal cord.

Between sum of squares Mathematical calculation involving the square of a number (i.e. the number multiplied by itself). 'Between sum' is the difference of the summation of two or more sets of numbers.

Bit Abbreviation of BInary digiT. Smallest unit of information: a single digit (0 or 1) in computing language.

Brainstem Enlarged extension upwards within the skull of the spinal cord, consisting of the medulla oblongata, the pons, and the midbrain.

Bruxism Tooth grinding: see Temporomandibular Joint Syndrome.

Cardiovascular system Heart together with two networks of blood vessels: systemic circulation, pulmonary circulation.

Causal correlation When there are two events, the presence of one event is the cause of the second event [e.g. an increase (or decrease) in rain causes an increase (or decrease) in the growth rate of grass]. Both events may be the cause of each other.

Cerebellar inco-ordination Connections of nerves in cerebellum of the brain not working sequentially or in union.

Cerebellar system Connections of nerves in cerebellum of the brain.

Cerebral aneurysm Balloon-like swelling in wall of an artery in the brain, due to disease or congenital deficiency.

Cerebral palsy Developmental abnormality of brain often caused by injury during birth resulting in weakness and inco-ordination of limbs.

Cerebrovascular accident Lesion or blockage in blood vessels of one or both hemispheres of the brain. Also known as 'stroke'.

Coccyx The lowermost element of the backbone: the vestigial human tail. Consists of four rudimentary coccygeal vertebrae fused to form a triangular bone that articulates with the sacrum.

Cognitive Style Psychological term. Assumed covert mental attitude.

Collateral blood supply Channels of communication between blood vessels supplying the heart.

Computerized tomography X-ray scanner incorporating computer, used to provide an integrated 3–D image of the soft structures of the body, particularly the brain. It can reveal presence of tumours, fluid, etc.

Conditional probability formulae Formulae used to express the probability of an event conditional on the probabilities of one or more other events (e.g. that used to derive Bayes' Theorem).

Contracture Fibrosis of muscle tissue producing shrinkage and shortening of muscle without generating any strength.

Contralateral Belonging to or occurring on opposite side of the body.

Corpus Callosum Broad band of nervous tissue that connects the two cerebral hemispheres.

Correlation Mutual relationship, (measure of extent of) inter-dependence of variable quantities, act of correlating.

Cortical Controlled by the cortex (outer grey area) of the brain.

Cranial nerves The twelve pairs of nerves that arise directly from the brain and leave the skull through separate apertures.

Cranial vessels Blood vessels of the skull.

Decubitus The recumbent position.

Decubitus ulcer An ulcerated area of the skin caused by irritation and continuous pressure on part of the body in a bedridden patient.

Deltoid Thick triangular muscle that covers the shoulder joint. Responsible for abduction, flexion and extension of shoulder joint.

Dementia Chronic or persistent disorder of mental processes due to organic brain disease. Marked by memory disorders, changes in personality, deterioration in personal care, impaired reasoning ability and disorientation.

Discrete interval data Discontinuous data that can be organized according to a rule (e.g. an arbitrary scale of whole number values that are spaced evenly apart).

Distal joints Joints furthest from limb or trunk of body.

Dorsiflexion Flexion of ankle joint pointing toes up towards the front of the leg.

Dorsum Upper or posterior surface of a part of the body.

Dynamometer Elliptical ring of steel to which is attached a dial and moving index. Used to test strength of muscles, usually forearm, being squeezed in hand, and registering in pounds or kilograms.

Dysfunction Impairment or abnormality of functioning of an organ.

Dyslexia Developmental disorder selectively affecting a child's ability to learn to read and write. Sometimes called specific dyslexia or developmental dyslexia to distinguish it from acquired difficulties with reading and writing.

Dysmetria Sometimes termed past-pointing. Attempt at touching object with finger results in overshooting object to one side. This promptly initiates a gross corrective action, but the correction overshoots to the other side. Consequently, the finger oscillates back and forth, and the further it travels, the greater the excursions become. This oscillation is the intention tremor of cerebellar disease.

Dysphagia Condition in which action of swallowing is either difficult to perform, painful, or in which swallowed material seems to be held up in its passage to the stomach.

EEG Electroencephalogram.

Efferent Designating nerves or neurones that convey impulses from the brain or spinal cord to muscles, glands, and other effectors (e.g. gamma efferents).

Electrocardiogram A recording of electrical activity of heart on moving paper strip. Tracing recorded by means of an electro-cardiograph.

Electrode Part of electrical conductor or recording device used to collect electrical activity from e.g. the heart or the brain.

Electroencephalography Study of electrical activity of the brain.

Electrogonimetric feedback Electrical feedback of joint angle of limbs.

Electromyography Study of electrical activity in muscles.

Embolism Obstruction of artery, etc. by clot of blood, air bubble, etc. especially as cause of paralysis. Clot may move from site; treatment by anticoagulant therapy.

EMG Electromyograph.

Engram Memory-trace, supposed permanent change in brain accounting for existence of memory.

Equilibrium Balance.

Eversion Turning outward.

Excursion Deviation of limb from regular path of movement.

Extensor Any muscle that causes straightening of limb or other part.

Exteroceptive stimuli Stimuli from outside the body detected by sensory nerve (exteroceptor), ending in the skin or a mucous membrane.

Facilitation of spontaneous movements Stimulation of spontaneous movement reactions, including righting and equilibrium reactions, in response to special techniques of handling the patient.

Facilitation of voluntary movements Achieved by positioning the patient in preparation for specific voluntary movements as certain movements are easier to perform from certain postural sets.

Fibrosis Thickening and scarring of connective tissue, most often a consequence of inflammation or injury.

Firing patterns Sequence of nerve impulses.

Flaccidity A decrease in muscle tone (e.g. in femoral paralysis).

Flexion Bending of one part of the body towards another usually towards ventral surface.

Flexor Any muscle that causes bending of limb or other part.

Frontal lobe Anterior part of each cerebral hemisphere, extending as far back as the deep central sulcus of its upper and outer surface.

Frontalis Muscle of the frontal bone (forehead).

Gait Manner of walking.

Glenoid fossa Socket of the shoulder joint: the pear-shaped cavity at the top of the scapula into which the head of the humerus fits.

Haemorrhage Escape of blood from blood vessels.

Hamstring Any tendons at the back of knee. Hamstring muscles are: biceps femoris, semitendinosus and semimembranosus, attached by hamstrings to their insertions in the tibia and fibula.

Handling Refers to techniques of holding and moving the patient in a way that will influence postural tone and regulate co-ordination of muscles.

Hardware The collective name for physical units comprising a computer.

Hemianaesthesia Loss of feeling or sensation in a part (one side) of the body.

Hemianopia Absence of half of the normal field of vision.

Hemiplegia A disorder of the Central Nervous System in which there is impairment of motor function and sensation on one side of the body.

Hemisphere One of the two halves of the cerebrum, not in fact hemispherical but more nearly quarter-spherical.

Holistic Approach to patient care in which physical, mental and social factors in the patient's condition are taken into account, rather than just the diagnosed disease.

Homolateral On or affecting the same side of the body.

Humerus Bone of the upper arm. Head of the humerus articulates with the scapula at the shoulder joint. At the lower end of the shaft the trochlea articulates with the ulna and part of the radius.

Hyperpyrexia Rise in body temperature above 41.1°C.

Hypertonicity (spasticity) Overactive muscular tonus.

Hypotonia (flaccidity) Abnormal decrease in muscle tension. May prevent maintenance of posture against gravity.

Infusion rate Slow injection of substance (e.g. saline or dextrose) into vein or subcutaneous tissue.

Inhibition Special techniques of handling aimed at reducing the hypertonic or athetoid patterns which prevent or interfere with normal muscle activity.

Input data file Set of data presented to a computer by devices such as keyboard, a second computer, specialized peripherals (e.g. joystick).

Insertion Point of attachment of a muscle (e.g. to a bone) that is relatively moveable when the muscle contracts.

Intention tremor May affect one limb or whole body. Gait is unsteady and whole arm comes into play when any attempt is made to use hand.

Interfacing Place, or piece of equipment, where interaction occurs between two systems, processes, etc.

Interphalangeal joint Joint between phalanges (i.e. finger and toes).

Intracerebral Within the cerebrum.

Intracerebral haemorrhage Escape of blood from ruptured blood vessel within brain.

Introspection Examine one's own thoughts and feelings.

Ipsilateral Belonging to or occurring on same side of body.

Isokinetic Equal movement.

Isometric contraction Induced in muscles that are used when a limb is made to pull or push against something that does not move.

Isotonic contraction Contraction of muscles that have equal tonicity.

Kinesthesia The sense that enables the brain to be constantly aware of the position and movement of muscles in different parts of the body.

Limb load monitor Device for monitoring load capabilities of individual limbs for correcting static limb loading patterns. Krusen LLM is an aid for gait training.

Local muscular phenomenon Isolated muscles are responsible.

Localized muscle fatigue Reduction in efficiency of isolated muscles.

Medial gastrocnemius Mid-line posterior (calf) muscle behind the tibia.

Motor ataxia Impairment in co-ordination of muscles.

Motor deficit Loss of neuromuscular power.

Motor neurone One of the units making up the nerve pathway between the brain and an effector organ, such as a skeletal muscle.

Motor performance Neuromuscular action.

Motor unit (recruitment) Nerve connections responsible for performing movement of muscles.

Multiple sclerosis Chronic disease of nervous system affecting young and middle-aged. Myelin sheaths surrounding nerves in brain and spinal cord are damaged, which effects function of nerves involved. Course of illness characterized by recurrent relapses followed by remissions. Symptoms include ataxia and spastic weakness.

Muscle action potential Nerve impulses across muscle fibres.

Myelin sheath Lipoid substance around some nerve fibres.

Myocardial infarction Death of segment of heart muscle, which follows interruption of its blood supply. Sudden severe pain, which may spread to arms and throat.

Myoelectrical potential Electrical activity of muscle.

Neurone Nerve cell, including its processes.

Nystagmus Rapid involuntary movements of the eyes that may be from side to side, up and down, or rotatory. May be congenital and associated with poor sight; it also occurs in disorders of the part of the brain responsible for eye movements and in disorders of the organ of balance in the ear.

Ontogeny The history of the development of an individual from the fertilized egg to maturity.

Operant conditioning Psychological term. Method of shaping behaviour by modifying and reinforcing successive responses. Sometimes responses are unexpected or undesired and may require considerable modification before the desired outcome is achieved.

Origin End of muscle that is ordinarily the fixed end.

Orthotic Concerned with splinting or bracing.

Pacinian corpuscles Sensory receptors for touch in the skin, consisting of sensory nerve-endings surrounded by capsules of membrane. They are especially sensitive to changes in pressure and so detect vibration particularly well.

Palpation Process of examining part of the body by careful feeling with the hands and fingertips.

Parasympathetic nervous system One of the two divisions of the autonomic nervous system, having fibres that leave the Central Nervous System from the brain and lower portion of the spinal cord and are distributed to blood vessels, glands, and internal organs. The nerve endings release acetylcholine as a neurotransmitter.

Paresthesia Abnormal tingling sensation: 'pins and needles'.

Parietal lobe One of the major divisions of each cerebral hemisphere, lying beneath the crown of the skull. Contains the sensory cortex and association areas.

Parkinsonism Disorder of middle-aged and elderly, characterized by tremor, rigidity and a poverty of spontaneous movements.

Passive stretch Assisted muscular stretch usually by therapists during assessment.

Patterns of movement The co-ordinated synergic actions of muscle groups that occur in normal movement and postural change.

Phalanges Segments of limb such as the fingers and toes.

Phylogeny Evolution of animal or plant type.

Placebo effect Psychological phenomenon in which the outcome of treatment is the same in the absence of a drug or technique as it is with the drug or technique.

Plantar reflex Reflex obtained by drawing a bluntly-pointed object along the outer border of the sole of the foot. The normal response is a bunching and downward movement of the toes.

Plethysmography Measurement of changes in the volume of a limb due to alterations in blood pressure, using an oncometer.

Poliomyelitis Infectious viral inflammation of nerve cells in grey matter of spinal cord, with temporary or permanent paralysis.

Prognosis Forecast of course of the disease.

Prone Lying with face downwards. Of the forearm: palm of hand faces downwards.

Proprioception Relating to stimuli produced and perceived within the organism (i.e. internal body awareness).

Proximal joints Joints nearest attached-end of limb or the trunk of the body.

RAM Random access memory – computer memory normally inside a computer as opposed to external memory such as discs.

Ramus Branch, especially of a nerve fibre or blood vessel.

Reflex inhibiting postures and patterns of movement These are postures and patterns of movement used to break up pathological reflex activity.

Resting potential When a neurone is not conducting impulses the inner surface of its plasma membrane is slightly negative – typically about -70mV – to its outer surface. This potential difference across a non-conducting neurone's plasma membrane is called the resting potential.

Reticular activating system Consists of centres in the brainstem reticular formation plus fibres that conduct to the centres from below and fibres that conduct from the centres to widespread areas of the cerebral cortex. Functioning is essential for consciousness.

Reticular formation Network of nerve pathways and nuclei throughout the brainstem, connecting motor and sensory nerves to and from the spinal cord, the cerebellum and the cerebrum, and the cranial nerves.

Rigidity A form of hypertonicity in which there is resistance to passive movement throughout a range of motion. Can be generalized resulting in very stiff posture and movement.

Segment Portion of tissue or organ, usually distinguishable from the others by lines of demarcation. Segment of a limb (e.g. toe, finger).

Software All programs that can be used on a particular computer.

Somatic Relating to the body rather than the mind.

Spasticity All the muscles in limb or limbs are hypertonic, and most powerful groups pull joints into positions of deformity.

Spastic resistance Resistance of muscle to movement due to spasticity.

Spindle A collection of fibres seen in a cell when it is dividing.

Stereognosis Ability to recognize the 3–D shape of an object by touch alone. This is a function of the association areas of the parietal lobe of the brain.

Stochastic model Method of prediction by laws of probability.

Subarachnoid haemorrhage Bleeding into the subarachnoid space that causes severe headache with stiffness of the neck. Usual source of such a haemorrhage is a cerebral aneurysm that has burst.

Subarachnoid space Space between the arachnoid and pia meninges of the brain and spinal cord, containing cerebro-spinal fluid and large blood vessels.

Supine Lying on the back with the face upwards. Of the forearm: the palm of the hand faces upwards.

Supraspinal Over or above the spinal column.

Sympathetic nervous system One of the two divisions of the autonomic nervous system, having fibres that leave the Central Nervous System in the thoratic and lumbar regions and are distributed to the blood vessels, sweat glands, salivary glands, heart, lungs, intestines and other abdominal organs. The nerve endings release noradrenaline as a neurotransmitter.

Synapse Minute gap across which nerve impulses pass from one neurone to the next, at the end of a nerve fibre. Reaching a synapse, an impulse causes the release of a neurotransmitter, which diffuses across the gap and triggers an electric impulse in the next neurone.

Synergist Muscle that acts with a prime mover (agonist) in making a particular movement.

Synkinesis With movement; tactile. Connected with or perceived by the sense of touch.

Temporomandibular Joint Syndrome Myofacial-pain-dysfunction-syndrome resulting from chronic clenching of the temporomandibular joint. Sufferers utilize their jaw musculature inappropriately when involved in tasks of a general nature. Syndrome is marked by limitations of mandibular movement, deviation of mandible on opening, clicking or crepitis of joint, dislocation, ringing in the ears, bruxism.

Thrombosis Condition in which the blood changes from a liquid to a solid state and produces a stationary blood clot (thrombus). Thrombosis in an artery obstructs the blood flow to the tissue it supplies.

Tibialis-anterior Muscle which dorsiflexes the ankle joint.

Tibio-tarsic isometric torque Movement of system of muscular forces tending to cause rotation at the top of foot during non-contraction (i.e. when the muscles are caused to act against each other or against a fixed object).

Torque Movement of system of muscular forces tending to cause rotation.

Torso Trunk of human stature apart from head and limbs.

Torticollis Also called wry neck. Rheumatic disease of muscle of neck causing twisting and stiffness.

Tumour Local swelling especially from morbid or abnormal growth; may be benign or malignant.

Vascular Consisting of vessels or ducts conveying blood.

References

Adams, G.F., Hurwitz, L.J. (1963) Mental barriers to recovery from strokes, *Lancet*, **ii**: 533–7.

Adler, M.K., Brown, C.C. and Acton, P. (1980) Stroke rehabilitation – Is age a determinant?, *Journal of the American Geriatric Society*, **28**, no. 11, 499–503.

Aho, K., Harmsen, P., Hatano, S., Marquardsen, J., Smirnov, V.E. *et al.* (1980) Cerebrovascular disease in the community: Results of a collaborative study, *Bull. WHO*, **58**, 113–30.

Alexander, A.B., French, C.A. and Goodman, N.J. (1975) A comparison of audio and visual feedback in biofeedback assisted muscular relaxation training, *Psychophysiology*, **12**, 119–23.

Allen, C.M.C. (1984a) Predicting outcome after acute stroke: Role of computerised tomography, *Lancet*, **ii**, 464–5.

Allen, C.M.C. (1984b) Clinical diagnosis of stroke, *Lancet*, **i**, 1357.

Allen, C.M.C. (1984c) Predicting outcome after acute stroke: A prognostic score, *Lancet*, **47**, 475–80.

Amato, A., Hermsmeyer, C.A. and Kleinman, K.M. (1973) Use of electromyographic feedback to increase inhibitory control of spastic muscles, *Physical Therapy*, **53**, 1063–6.

An, K.N., Chao, E. and Asken, L.J. (1980) Hand strength measurement instruments, *Archives in Physical Medicine Rehabilitation*, **61**, 366.

Arsenault, A.B. and Chapman, A.E. (1974) An electromyographic examination of the individual recruitment of the quadriceps muscles during isometric contraction of the knee extensors in different patterns of movement, *Physiotherapy of Canada*, **26**, no. 5, 253–61.

Arthur, C. (1986) Who pays if you dial D for diagnosis but end up with death? *Computer Weekly*, **10**, no. 1, 28.

Ashley, M.J. (1982) Alcohol consumption, ischaemic heart disease and cerebrovascular disease, *Journal of Studies on Alcohol*, **43**, 869–87.

Assael, H. (1970) Segmenting markets by group purchasing behaviour: An application of the AID technique, *Journal of Marketing Research*, **vii**, 153–8.

Bach-y-Rita, P. (1980) *Recovery of Function: Theoretical Considerations for Brain Injury Rehabilitation*, University Park Press, Baltimore.

Bach-y-Rita, P. (1981) Brain plasticity as a basis for the development of rehabilitation procedures for hemiplegia, *Scandinavian Journal of Rehabilitation Medicine*, **13**, 73–3.

Baker, L., Yeh, C., Wilson, D. and Waters, R.L. (1979) Electrical stimulation of hemiplegic hand for treatment of contractures, *Archives in Physical Medicine Rehabilitation*, **60**, no. 11, 497–502.

Balliet, R., Levy, B. and Blood, K.M.T. (1986) Upper extremity sensory feedback therapy in chronic cerebrovascular accident patients with impaired expressive aphasia and auditory comprehension, *Archives in Physical Medicine Rehabilitation*, **67**, no. 5, 304–10.

REFERENCES

Banks, G.B., Caplan, L.R. and Hier, D.B. (1983) The Michael Reese Stroke Registry: A microcomputer-implemented database, *Proceedings of the 7th Annual Symposium of Computer Applications in Medical Care*, 724-7.

Barker, P.G. (1984) MICROTEXT: A new dialogue programming language for microcomputers, *Journal of Microcomputer Applications*, 7, 167-88.

Barker, P.G. and Singh, R. (1983) A practical introduction to authoring for computer-assisted instruction. Part 2. PILOT, *British Journal of Education Technology*, 14, no. 3, 174-200.

Barker, P.G. and Steele, J. (1983) A practical introduction to authoring for computer assisted instruction. Part 1: IPS, *British Journal of Education Technology*, 14, no. 1, 26-45.

Barnford, J., Sandercock, P., Warlow, C. and Gray, M. (1986) Why are patients with acute stroke admitted to hospital? *British Medical Journal*, 292, 1369-72.

Basmajian, J.V. (1963) Control and training of individual motor units, *Science*, 141, 440-1.

Basmajian, J.V. (1967) Control of individual motor units, *American Journal of Physical Medicine*, 46, 480-6.

Basmajian, J.V. (1981) Biofeedback in rehabilitation: A review of principles and practices, *Archives in Physical Medicine Rehabilitation*, 62, no. 10, 469-75.

Basmajian, J.V., Kulkulka, B.S., Narayan, M.D. and Takeb, M.D. (1975) Biofeedback treatment of foot-drop after stroke compared with standard rehabilitation technique: Effects on voluntary control and strength, *Archives in Physical Medicine Rehabilitation*, 56, 231-6.

Bazzini, G., Guarnaschelli, C., Casale, R. and Zelaschi, F. (1984) Studio di un feedback visivo sul momento massimo volontario di flessione dorsale della tibiotarsica in pazienti emplegici, *Bollettino della Societa Italiano Biologia Speriment'ale*, 60, no. 2, 375-81.

Beilin, L.J., Bullpitt, C.J., Coles, E.C., Dollery, C.T., Johnson, B.F. *et al.* (1974) Computer-based hypertension clinic records: A cooperative study, *British Medical Journal*, 2, 212-6.

Birnbaum, I. (1984) Framing the right questions, *Acorn User*, 10, 137-41.

Blanchard, E.B. and Young, L.D. (1972) Relative efficacy of visual and auditory feedback for self-control of heart rate, *Journal of General Psychology*, 87, 195-202.

Bobath, B. (1959) Observations on adult hemiplegia and suggestions for treatment, *Physiotherapy*, 12.

Bobath, B. (1964) The facilitation of normal postural reactions and movements in the treatment of cerebral palsy, *Physiotherapy*, 8, 3-9.

Bobath, B. (1967) The very early treatment of cerebral palsy, *Developmental Medicine in Child Neurology*, 9, no. 4, 373-90.

Bobath, B. (1969) The treatment of neuromuscular disorders by improving patterns of coordination, *Physiotherapy*, 1.

Bobath, B. (1971) *Abnormal Postural Reflex Activity Caused by Brain Lesions*, Heinemann, London.

Bobath, B. (1977) Treatment of adult hemiplegia, *Physiotherapy*, 63, no. 10, 310-3.

Bobath, B. (1985) *Adult Hemiplegia: Evaluation and Treatment*, Heinemann, London.

Bolton, L. (1985) A picture of health, *Computing*, **11**, no. 1, 9–10.

Booth, K. (1982) The neglect syndrome, *Journal of Neurosurgical Nursing*, **14**, 38–43.

Borden, W.A. (1962) Psycho-social aspects of stroke patient and family, *Annals of International Medicine*, **57**, 689.

Borello-France, D.F., Burdett, R.G. and Gee, Z.L. (1988) Modification of sitting posture of patients with hemiplegia using seat boards and back boards, *Physical Therapy*, **68**, no. 1, 67–71.

Bowman, B.R., Baker, L.L. and Waters, R. (1979) Positional feedback and electrical stimulation: An automated treatment for the hemiplegic wrist, *Archives in Physical Medicine Rehabilitation*, **60**, 497–502.

Boyd, R.V. (1987) The rehabilitation of stroke illness, *The Practitioner*, **231**, no. 6, 890–5.

Brunnström, S. (1956) Associated reactions of the upper extremity in adult patients with hemiplegia. An approach to training, *Physical Therapy Review*, **36**, 225–36.

Brunnström, S. (1962) Training the hemiplegic patient: Orientation of techniques to patient's motor behaviour, in *Approach to the Treatment of Patients with Neuromuscular Dysfunction* (ed. C. Satterley), William Brown, Iowa, pp. 44–8.

Brunnström, S. (1966) Motor testing procedures in hemiplegia based on recovery stages, *JAPTA*, **46**, 357–75.

Brunnström, S. (1970) *Movement Therapy in Hemiplegia*, Harper and Row, New York.

Brunnström, S. (1971) Motor behaviour of adult hemiplegic patients, *American Journal of Occupational Therapy*, **XXV**, no. 1, 6–12.

Brzoza, R., Janota, B. and Wolniczek, B. (1981) Zastosowanie metod zastepczego sprzezenia zwrotnego w usprawnieniu chodu chorych po udarach mozgowych, *Wiad Lek*, **34**, no. 6, 481–6.

Buzzi, R. and Battig, K. (1983) Computerized recording of multichannel biological functions, in *Advances in Biosciences Vol. 46 – Neuro-Behavioural Methods in Occupational Health*, (eds R. Gilioli, M.G. Cassitto and V. Foa), Pergamon, Oxford, pp. 148–55.

Cassell, K., Shaw, K. and Stern, G.A. (1973) A computerised tracking technique for assessment of parkinsonian motor disabilities, *Brain*, **96**, 815–26.

Chapman, N.W. (1986) The Hospital and Health Service Year Book 1986, *London Institute of Health Services Management*.

Chernikova, L.A. (1984) Method elektromiograficheskoi obratnoi sviazi v komple-ksnom vosstanovitel'nom lechenii bol'nykh s postinsul'tnymidvi gatel'nymi rasstroistvami, *Zhurnal Nevropatologii i Psikhiatrii*, **84** 12, 1795–8.

Chessington Occupational Therapy Neurological Assessment Battery: available from Nottingham Rehab., Ludlow Hill Rd, West Brigford, Notts, NG2 6HD.

Coe, F., Norton, E., Oparil, S. and Pullman, T.N. (1975) Physician acceptance of computer recommended antihypertensive therapy, *Computers in Biomedical Research*, **8**, 492–502.

Cohen, B.A., Bravo-Fernandez, E.J. and Sances, A. Jr. (1976a) Application of automated analysis of serial electroencephalograms for stroke prognosis, *29th Annual Conference on Engineering in Medicine and Biology*, **12**, no. 11, 223.

Cohen, B.A., Bravo-Fernandez, E.J. and Sances, A. Jr. (1976b) Quantification of computer analysed serial EEGs from stroke patients, *Electroencephalography and Clinical Neurophysiology*, **41**, no. 4, 379–86.

Coleman, M.J. (1984) *Disk Programming Techniques for the BBC Microcomputer*, Prentice-Hall International, London.

Coll, J. (1982) *The BBC Microcomputer User Guide*, British Broadcasting Corporation, London.

Collin, M.E. (1973) An analytical study of selected neurophysiological techniques suggesting their relevance in occupational therapy, *A Dissertation Presented to the Faculty of Medicine*, Witwatersrand University.

Collin, M.E. (1975) Neurophysiological techniques in the treatment of adult neurologically impaired patients, *British Journal of Occupational Therapy*, **8**, 166–7.

Collin, S.J., Tinson, D. and Lincoln, N.B. (1987) Depression after stroke, *Clinical Rehabilitation*, **1**, 27–32.

Coxon, A.P.M. (1982) *The Users' Guide to Multidimensional Scaling*, Heinemann, London.

Cressman, M.D. and Gifford, R.W. (1983) Hypertension and stroke, *Journal of American Coll. and Cardiology*, **1**, 521–7.

Crofts, F. and Crofts, J. (1988) Biofeedback and the computer, *British Journal of Occupational Therapy*, **51**, no. 2, 57–9.

Danniels, L. and Worthington, C. (1972) *Testing Techniques of Manual Examination*, Saunders, Philadelphia.

Davies, B. and Knapp, M. (1986) A treatment for the hemiplegic arm. *British Journal of Occupational Therapy*, **49**, no. 7, 225–6.

Davies, P.M. (1985) *Steps to Follow: A Guide to the Treatment of Adult Hemiplegia*, Springer-Verlag, New York.

Davis, A.E. and Lee, R.G. (1980) EMG biofeedback in patients with motor disorders: An aid for coordinating activity in antagonistic muscle groups, *Canadian Journal of Neurological Science*, **7**, no. 3, 199–206.

Demidenko, T.D., L'vova, R.I., Inin Ius., Iakovlev, N.M. and Bogdanov, O.V. (1983) Primenie portativnykh biotekhnicheskikh ustroistv sobratnoi sviaz'iu v sistemeaktivnoi vosstanovitel'noi terapii u bol'nykh s postinsul'tnymi dvigatel'nymi narusheniiami, *Zhurnal Nevropatologii i Psikhiatrii*, **83**, no. 8, 1121–6.

Dennis, M.S. and Warlow, C.P. (1987) Stroke – incidence, risk factors and outcome, *British Journal of Hospital Medicine*, **3**, 194–8.

De Souza, L.H., Langton-Hewer, R. and Miller, S. (1980) 1: Assessment of recovery of arm control in hemiplegic stroke patients. The arm function test, *International Rehabilitation Medicine*, **2**, no. 1, 3.

Doerr, J.A., Estes, J.T. and Tourtellotte, W.W. (1977) Portable clinical tracking task equipment, *Medical Biological and Engineering Computing*, **15**, 391–7.

Doyle, P. and Fenwick, I. (1975) The pitfalls of AID analysis, *Journal of Marketing Research*, **xii**, 408–13.

Driscoll, M.C. (1975) Creative technological aids for the learning-disabled child, an interdisciplinary project, *American Journal of Occupational Therapy*, **29**, 102–5.

Drummond, A.E.R. (1988) Stroke: The impact on the family, *British Journal of Occupational Therapy*, **51**, no. 6, 193–4.

Dzierzanowski, J.M., Bourne, J.R., Shiavi, R., Sandell, H.S.H. and Guy, D. (1985) GAITSPERT: An expert system for the evaluation of abnormal human locomotion arising from stroke, *IEEE*, **32**, no. 11, 935–42.

Ebrahim, S. (1985) Depression after stroke: A common cause of rehabilitation failure, *Geriatric Medicine*, **15**, no. 7, 5–6.

Ediss, P.B. and Grove, E. (1983) Microcomputers in Occupational Therapy departments of hospitals and day centres, *British Journal of Occupational Therapy*, **46**, no. 8, 222.

Editorial (1983) 'Binge' drinking and stroke, *Lancet*, **ii**, 223–6.

Edmans, J.A. (1987) *Handbook for Rehabilitation of Stroke Patients*, available from Occupational Therapy Department, General Hospital, Nottingham.

Edmans, J.A. and Lincoln, N.B. (1987) The frequency of perceptual deficits after stroke, *Clinical Rehabilitation*, **1**, 273–81.

Eggers, O. (1983) *Occupational Therapy in the Treatment of Adult Hemiplegia*, Heinemann, London.

Ellenberg, J. (1977) Minutes of task force meeting to evaluate need for stroke data bank model, *Report of National Institute of Neurological Communicative Disorders and Stroke*, Washington DC.

Feigenson, J.S. (1976) Stroke rehabilitation: Factors influencing outcome and length of stay, *Archives in Physical Medicine Rehabilitation*, **57**, 530–1.

Feigenson, J.S., Fries, J.F., Kunitz, S., McShane, D. and Greenberg, S.D. (1979a) Time-orientated functional profile: Practical application in a stroke database model, *Archives in Physical Medicine Rehabilitation*, **60**, 512–6.

Feigenson, J.S. and Greenberg, S.D. (1979) Disability oriented stroke unit; Major factors influencing stroke outcomes, *Stroke*, **10**, 5–8.

Feigenson, J.S. and McCarthy, M.L. (1977) Stroke rehabilitation II: Guidelines for establishing stroke rehabilitation unit, *New York State Journal of Medicine*, **77**, 1430–4.

Feigenson, J.S., McCarthy, M.L., Greenberg, S.D., Feigenson, W.D. and Rubin, E. (1977) Factors influencing outcome and length of stay in stroke rehabilitation unit. Part 2: Comparison of 318 screened and 248 unscreened patients, *Stroke*, **8**, 657–62.

Feigenson, J.S., McCarthy, M.L. and Meese, P.D. (1977) Stroke rehabilitation I: Factors predicting outcome and length of stay – an overview, *New York State Journal of Medicine*, **8**, 1426–30.

Feigenson, J.S., McCarthy, M.L., Polkow, L., Meikle, R. and Ferguson, W. (1979b) Burke Stroke Time-Oriented Profile (BUSTOP): An overview of patient function, *Archives of Physical Medicine Rehabilitation*, **60**, 508–11.

Felsenthal, G. (1982a) An overview of clinical application of electromyography and nerve conduction techniques. Part 1: Electromyographic and nerve conduction techniques, *MD State Medical Journal*, **31**, 59–61.

REFERENCES

Felsenthal, G. (1982b) An overview of clinical application of electromyography and nerve conduction techniques. Part 2: Diagnostic applications, *MD State Medical Journal*, **31**, no. 10, 50–3.

Fernando, C.K. and Basmajian, J.V. (1978) Biofeedback in physical medicine and rehabilitation, *Biofeedback Self Regulation*, **3**, 435–50.

Fieschi, M., Joubert, M., Fieschi, D. and Roux, M. (1982) SPHINX: A system for computer-aided diagnosis, *Methodology and Information in Medicine*, **21**, 143–8.

Fisher, S.H. (1961) Psychiatric consideration of cerebral vascular disease, *American Journal of Cardiology*, **7**, 379.

Fix, E. and Neyman, J. (1951) A simple stochastic model of recovery, relapse, death and loss of patients, *Human Biology*, **23**, 205–41.

Fleischman, E.A. (1972) Structure and measurement of psychomotor abilities, in *The Psychomotor Domain* (ed. R.N. Singer), Lea and Febiger, Philadelphia, pp. 78–106.

Flowers, K.A. (1976) Visual 'closed loop' and 'open loop' characteristics of voluntary movement in patients with parkinsonianism and intention tremor, *Brain*, **99**, 269–310.

Fries, J.F. (1976) Editorial: A data bank for the clinician, *New England Journal of Medicine*, **294**, 1400–2.

Fugl-Meyer, A.R., Jaasko, L., Leiman, I., Olson, S. and Steglind, S. (1975) The post-stroke hemiplegic: A method for evaluation of physical performance, *Scandinavian Journal of Rehabilitation Medicine*, **61**, 13.

Gaudette, M., Prins, A. and Kahane, J. (1983) Comparison of auditory and visual feedback for EMG trainings, *Perceptual Motor Skills*, **56**, 383–6.

Gelman, J., Lakie, M., Walsh, E.G. and Wright, G.W. (1978) Treatment of hemiplegia by feedback induced muscular exercise, *Journal of Physiology*, **285**, 6P–7P.

Gentry, W.D., Jenkins, C.D., Caplan, P.H., Hayman, A., Breslin, M.S. *et al.* (1979) Type A behaviour pattern and ischaemic cerebrovascular disease, *Heart and Lung*, **8**, 1113–6.

Gill, J.S., Zezulka, A.V. and Shipley, M.J. (1986) Stroke: New link to heavy alcohol consumption, *New England Journal of Medicine*, **315**, 1041–6.

Goetter, W. (1986) Nursing diagnoses and interventions with the acute stroke patient, *Nursing Clinical of North America*, **21**, no. 2, 309–19.

Goldberg, S. (1983) *Clinical Neuroanatomy Made Ridiculously Simple*, Medmaster Inc.

Gresham, G.E. (1986) Stroke outcome research, *Stroke*, **17**, no. 3, 358–9.

Gretton, S. (1986) The foundations and practice of sensory-motor therapy, in *Therapy Through Movement*, (ed. L.A. Burr) Nottingham Rehab. Ltd, pp 3–53.

Gruskin, A.K., Abitante, S.M. and Gorski, A.T. (1983) Auditory feedback device in a patient with left-sided neglect, *Archives in Physical Medicine Rehabilitation*, **64**, no. 12, 606–7.

Hards, B., Thompson, S.B.N. and Bate, R. (1986) A program of therapeutic interest, *Therapy Weekly*, **12**, no. 31, 7.

Harrison, M.J.G. and Dyken, M.L. (1983) *Cerebral Vascular Disease*, Butterworths, London.

Hart, G. (1983) Strokes causing left vs right hemiplegia: Different effects and nursing implications, *Geriatric Nursing*, **4**, 39–42.

Hay, E., Royds, J.A., Davies-Jones, G. *et al.* (1984) Cerebrospinal enolase in acute stroke, *Journal of Neurosurgical Psychiatry*, **47**, 724–9.

Heinemann, A.W., Eliot, J.R., Cichowski, K. and Betts, H.B. (1987) Multivariate analysis of improvement and outcome following stroke rehabilitation, *Archives of Neurology*, **44**, 1167–72.

Herman, B., Layten, A.C.M., van Luijk, J.H. *et al.* (1982a) An evaluation of risk factors for stroke in a Dutch community, *Stroke*, **13**, 334–9.

Herman, B., Layten, A.C.M., van Luijk, J.H. *et al.* (1982b) Epidemiology of stroke in Tilberg, the Netherlands, *Stroke*, **13**, 629–34.

Hertanu, J.S., Demopaulos, J.T., Yang, W.C., Calhoun, W.F., Fenigstein, O.T.R. (1984) Stroke rehabilitation: Correlation and prognostic value of computerised tomography and sequential functional assessments, *Archives in Physical Medicine Rehabilitation*, **65**, 505–8.

Hier, D.B., Atkinson, G.D., Perline, R. *et al.* (1986) Can a patient database help build a stroke diagnostic expert system? *Medical Information*, **11**, no. 1, 75–81.

Hill, G.L. and Smith, A.H. (1974) Buerger's disease in Indonesia: Clinical course and prognostic factors, *Journal of Chronic Diseases*, **27**, 205–16.

Hillbom, M. and Kaste, M. (1983) Ethanol intoxication: A risk for ischaemic brain infarction, *Stroke*, **14**, 694–9.

Hoskins, T. and Squires, J. (1973) Developmental assessment: A test for gross motor and reflex development, *Physical Therapy*, **53**, no. 2, 117–26.

Howe, J.R. (1977) *Patient Care in Neurosurgery*, Little, Brown and Co., Boston.

Hughes, E. (1972) Bobath and Brunnström. Comparison of two methods of treatment of a left hemiplegia, *Physiotherapy of Canada*, **24**, no. 5, 262–6.

Hume, C. (1984) Microcomputers in occupational therapy departments: The therapeutic application, *British Journal of Occupational Therapy*, **47**, no. 6, 175–7.

Hurd, S.N. (1975) Trends in treatment methods and media including the use of PNF and the Bobath approach. A survey of occupational therapy for the hemiplegic patient, *British Journal of Occupational Therapy*, **38**, no. 4, 81–3.

Huss, J. (1971) Sensorimotor treatment approaches, in *Occupational Therapy*, 4th edn, (eds Willard and Spackman) J.B. Lippincott Co., Philadelphia, pp. 380–3.

Hyland, M. (1981) *Introduction of Theoretical Psychology*, Macmillan, London.

Iosifescu, M. and Tautu, P. (1973) *Stochastic Processes and Applications in Biology and Medicine. II: Models*, Springer-Verlag, New York.

Isaacs, B. (1971) Identification of disability in the stroke patient, *Modern Geriatrics*, **9**, 390–403.

Isaacs, B. (1983) *Understanding Stroke Illness*, Chest, Heart and Stroke Association, London.

Isaacs, B., Neville, Y. and Rushford, I. (1976) The stricken: The social consequences of stroke, *Age and Ageing*, **5**, 188–92.

REFERENCES

Isaacs, B., Silverberg, N.E., Steven, R.C. and Schoening, H.A. (1979) Revised Kenny self-care evaluation, *Rehabilitation Publication 722*, Sister Kenny Institute, Minneapolis.

Iverson, J., Sproule, M., Leicht, M., Donald, W.M. and Campbell, D. (1976) Electromyographic biofeedback treatment of residual neuromuscular disabilities after cerebrovascular accident, *Physiotherapy of Canada*, **28**, 260–4.

Jansen, P.A.F., Schulte, B.P.M., Meyboom, R.H.B. and Gribnau, F.W.J. (1986) Antihypertensive treatment as a possible cause of stroke in the elderly, *Age and Ageing*, **15**, 129–38.

Jex, H.R., McDonnell, J.D. and Patah, A.V.A. (1986) 'Critical' tracking task for manual control research, *IEEE Transactions of Human Factor Electronics*, HFE–7, 138–45.

Johnson, H.E. and Garton, W.H. (1973) Muscle re-education in hemiplegia by use of electromyographic device, *Archives in Physical Medicine Rehabilitation*, **53**, 320–3.

Johnson, R., and Garvie, C. (1985) The BBC microcomputer for therapy of intellectual impairment following acquired brain damage, *British Journal of Occupational Therapy*, **48**, no. 2, 46–8.

Johnson, W.G. and Turin, A. (1987) Biofeedback treatment of migraine headache, *Behavioural Therapy*, **6**, 394–7.

Jones, R.D. (1975) The graphic display computer in rehabilitation, *New Zealand Medical Physics and Biomedical Engineering*, **2**, 5–10.

Jones, R.D. and Donaldson, I.M. (1981) Measurement of integrated sensory-motor function following brain damage by a computerised preview tracking task, *International Rehabilitation Medicine*, **3**, no. 2, 71–83.

Kannel, W.B. and Wolf, P.A. (1983) Epidemiology of cerebrovascular disease, *Vascular Disease of the Central Nervous System*, 2nd edn, (ed. R.W. Ross Russell), Churchill Livingstone, Edinburgh, pp. 1–24.

Kapur, N. (1984) Using a microcomputer-based data management system for neuropsychological record filing, report generation, and as a clinical aid, *Bulletin of the British Psychological Society*, **37**, 413–5.

Knott, M. (1973) In the groove, *Physical Therapy*, **53**, no. 4, 365–72.

Knott, M. and Voss, D.E. (1956) *Proprioceptive Neuromuscular Facilitation: Patterns, Techniques*, Hoeber Medical Division, Harper and Row, New York.

Koheil, R. and Mandel, A.R. (1980) Joint position biofeedback facilitation of physical therapy in gait training, *American Journal of Physical Medicine*, **59**, no. 6, 288–97.

Kwatny, E. and Zuckerman, R. (1975) Proceedings: Devices and systems for the disabled, *Report, Krusen Centre for Research and Engineering*, Moss Rehabilitation Hospitals, Philadelphia.

Lawrence, L. and Christie, D. (1979) Quality of life after stroke: A three year followup, *Age and Ageing*, **8**, 167–72.

Lee, K.H., Hill, E., Johnson, R. and Smiehorowski, T. (1976) Biofeedback for muscle retraining in hemiplegic patients, *Archives of Physical Medicine Rehabilitation*, **57**, 588–91.

Locheesoft OT/Remedial Software Series: available from Locheesoft Publications Ltd, Oak Villa, New Alyth, Blairgowrie, PH11 8NN, Scotland.

Logigian, M.K., Samuels, M.A., Falconer, J. and Zagar, R., (1983) Clinical exercise trial for stroke patients, *Archives in Physical Medicine Rehabilitation*, **64**, no. 5, 364–7.

Luciano, S.D., Vander, A.J. and Sherman, J.H. (1978) *Human Anatomy and Physiology: Structure and Function*, 2nd edn, McGraw-Hill, London.

Lynn, P.A., Reed, G.A., Parker, W.R. and Langton-Hewer, R. (1977) *Medical and Biological Engineering*, **15**, 184–8.

Mahoney, F.I. and Barthel, D.W. (1965) Functional evaluation: Barthel index, *MD State Medical Journal*, **14**, 61–5.

Marinacci, A.A. and Horande, M. (1960) Electromyogram in neuromuscular re-education, *Bulletin of the Los Angeles Neurological Society*, **25**, 57–71.

Marsh, R.W. (1980) Electromyographic feedback treatment of hemiplegia, *New Zealand Medical Journal*, **91**, no. 653, 96–7.

McSherry, D.M.G. and Fullerton, K.J. (1985) Preceptor: A shell for medical expert systems and its application in a study of prognostic indices in stroke, *Expert Systems*, **2**, no. 3, 140–7.

Miller, L.S. and Miyamato, A.T. (1979) Computed tompography: Its potential as predictor of functional recovery following stroke, *Archives in Physical Medicine Rehabilitation*, **60**, 108–9.

Mims, H.W. (1956) Electromyography in clinical practice, *Southern Medical Journal*, **49**, 804–6.

Morgan, M. (1986) Eating problems of the elderly, *Geriatric Nursing*, **6**, no. 6, 28–30.

Morgan, M. and Thompson S.B.N. (1989) Bridging the gap, *Therapy Weekly*, **15**, no. 40, 10.

Moskowitz, E. and McCann, C.B. (1967) Classification of disability in chronically ill and ageing, *Journal of Chronic Diseases*, **5**, 342–6.

Mroczek, N., Halpern, D. and McHugh, R. (1978) Electromyographic feedback and physical therapy for muscular retraining in hemiplegia, *Archives in Physical Medicine Rehabilitation*, **59**, 258–67.

Mykyta, L.J., Bowling, J.H., Nelson, D.A. and Lloyd, E.J. (1976) Caring for relatives of stroke patients, *Age and Ageing*, **5**, 87–90.

Newman, W.M. and Sproull, R.F. *Principles of Interactive Computer Graphics*, McGraw-Hill, London.

Ogg, H.L. (1963) Measuring and evaluating the gait patterns of children, *Journal of the American Physical Therapy Association*, **43**, 717–20.

Oxfordshire Community Stroke Project (1983) Incidence of stroke in Oxfordshire: First year's experience of a community stroke register, *British Medical Journal*, **287**, 713–6.

Parker, W.R., Reed, G.A., Baldwin, J.F. and Pilsworth, B.W. (1979) New approaches to modelling the disabled human operator, *Medical Biological Engineering Computing*, **17**, 344–8.

Perry, C.E. (1967) Principles and techniques of the Brunnström approach to the treatment of hemiplegia, *American Journal of Physical Medicine, NUSTEP Proceedings*, **46**, no. 1, 789–812.

Petherham, B. (1988) Enabling stroke victims to interact with a microcomputer – a comparison of input devices, *International Disability Studies*, **10**, 73–80.

REFERENCES

Pinelli, P. (1984) La riabilitazione neurologia del lavoratore emiplegico, *Giornale Italiano del Medico Lavorante*, **6**, 61–6.

Potvin, A.R. and Tourtellotte, W.W. (1975) The neurological examination: Advancements in its quantification, *Archives in Physical Medicine Rehabilitation*, **56**, 425–37.

Poulton, E.C. (1974) *Tracking Skill and Manual Control*, Academic Press, New York.

Raisman, G. and Field, P.M. (1973) A quantitative investigation of the development of collateral reinervation of the septal nuclei, *Brain Res.*, **50**, 241–64.

Reggia, J. (1982) Computer-assisted medical decision making, in *Applications of Computers in Medicine*, (ed. M. Schwartz), IEEE Press, Piscataw, New Jersey, pp. 198–213.

Rivermead Assessment Batteries for Activities of Daily Living, Perception, Memory and Unilateral Neglect available from Rivermead Rehabilitation Unit, Abingdon Rd; Oxford, OX1 4XD.

Rood, M. (1954) Neurophysiological reactions as a basis for physical therapy, *Physical Therapy Review*, **34**, no. 9, 66–7.

Rood, M. (1962) The use of sensory receptors to activate, facilitate and inhibit motor response, automatic and somatic, in developmental sequence, in *Approaches to the Treatment of Patients with Neuromuscular Dysfunction*, (ed. C. Sattely) William C. Brown, Dubuque, Iowa, pp. 36–7.

Rose, F. and Capildeo, R. (1981) *Stroke, The Facts*, Oxford University Press, New York.

Rosenberg, N.L. and Koller, R. (1981) Computerised tomography and pure sensory stroke, *Neurology (NY)*, **31**, no. 2, 217–20.

Ross Russell, R.W. (1983) *Vascular Disease of the Nervous System*, Churchill Livingstone, Edinburgh.

Rudy, E.B. (1984) *Advanced Neurological and Neurosurgical Nursing*, C.V. Mosby, St. Louis.

Ryan, E.D. (1962) Retention of stabilometer and pursuit rotor skills, *Research Quarterly*, **33**, 46–51.

Salamon, R., Bernadet, M. and Samson, M. (1976) Bayesian method applied to decision making in neurology. Methodological considerations, *Methods Inf. Med.*, **15**, 174–9.

Sandercock, P.A.G. (1984), *DM Thesis*, Oxford.

Savinelli, R., Timm, M., Montgomery, J., Wilson, D.J. (1978) Therapy evaluation and management of patients with hemiplegia, *Clin. Orthop.*, **31**, 15–29.

Schandler, S.L. and Grings, W.W. (1976) An examination of methods for producing relaxation during short-term laboratory sessions, *Behaviour, Research and Therapy*, **14**, 419–26.

Schmidt, R.A. (1975) *Motor Skills*, Harper and Row, New York.

Sell, P.S. (1985) *Expert Systems – A Practical Introduction*, Macmillan, Basingstoke.

Selley, W.G. (1985) Swallowing difficulties in stroke patients. A new treatment, *Age and Ageing*, **14**, 361–5.

Shafer, K.N., Sawyer, J.R., McCluskey, A.M., Beck, E.L. and Phipps, W.J. (1975) *Medical-Surgical Nursing*, C.V. Mosby, St. Louis.

Sharpless, J.W. (1982) *Mossman's Problem-Oriented Approach to Stroke Rehabilitation*, 2nd edn, Charles C. Thomas, Springfield.

Siev, E. and Freishstat, B. (1970) *Perceptual Dysfunction in Adult Stroke Patients*, Chas. B. Slack.

Sime, M.S. and Coombs, M.J. (1983) *Designing for Human-Computer Communication*, Academic Press, London.

Simpson, R.J. (1987) Remedial therapy referral times for stroke patients, *British Journal of Occupational Therapy*, **50**, no. 11, 379–80.

Skilbeck, C.E. (1984) Computer assistance in the management of memory and cognitive impairment, in *The Clinical Management of Memory Problems* (eds B. Wilson, M. Moffat), Croom Helm, London.

Smart, S. (1988) Computers as treatment: The use of the computer as an Occupational Therapy medium, *Clinical Rehabilitation*, **2**, 61–9.

Smith, A.H. (1975) *The Application of Stochastic Models in Chronic Disease Epidemiology*, PhD thesis, University of Otago, New Zealand.

Smith, A.H. (1978) The assessment of patient prognosis using an interactive computer program, *International Journal of Biomedical Computing*, **9**, no. 1, 37–44.

Sødring, K.M. (1980) The Bobath Concept in treatment of adult hemiplegia, *Scandinavian Journal of Rehabilitation Medicine (Supplement)*, **7**, 101–5.

Sonquist, J.A. (1970) *Multivariate Model Building*, University of Michigan, Institute for Social Research, Ann Arbor, Michigan.

Sonquist, J.A., Baker, E.L. and Morgan, J.N. (1971) *Searching for Structure (Alias AID – III)*, University of Michigan, Institute for Social Research, Ann Arbor, Michigan.

Sonquist, J.A., Baker, E.L. and Morgan, J.N. (1973) *Searching for Structure: An Approach to Substantial Bodies of Micro-Data and Documentation for a Computer Program*, University of Michigan, Institute for Social Research, Ann Arbor, Michigan.

Spearing, D.L. and Poppen, R. (1974) The use of feedback in the reduction of foot dragging in a cerebral palsied client, *J. Nerv. Ment. Dis.*, **159**, 148–51.

Spiegelhalter, D.J. and Knill-Jones, R.P. (1984) Statistical knowledge-based approaches to clinical decision-support systems, with an application in gastroenterology, *Journal of the Royal Statistics Society*, **147**, 35–77.

SPSS Inc. (1986) *SPSS–X User Guide*, 2nd edn, McGraw-Hill, New York.

Stanic, U., Acimovic-Janezic, R., Gross, N, *et al.* (1978) Multichannel electrical stimulation for correction of hemiplegic gait – methodology and preliminary results, *Scandinavian Journal of Rehabilitation Medicine*, **10**, 75–92.

Starmer, C.F., Rosati, R.A. and McNeer, J.F. (1974a) Data bank use in management of chronic disease, *Computers in Biomedical Research*, **7**, 111–6.

Starmer, C.F., Rosati, R.A. and McNeer, J.F. (1974b) A comparison of frequency distributions for use in a model for selecting treatment in coronary artery disease, *Computers in Biomedical Research*, **7**, 278–93.

Steed, A. (1986) Using the Steed cushion in the treatment of flaccid hemiplegia, *British Journal of Occupational Therapy*, **49**, no. 2, 34–8.

Stevens, R.S. and Amber, N.R. (1982) The incidence and survival of stroke patients in a defined community, *Age and Ageing*, **11**, 266–74.

Stockmeyer, S. (1967) An interpretation of the approach of Rood to the treatment of neuromuscular dysfunction, *American Journal of Physical Medicine, NUSTEP proceedings*, **46**, no. 1, 900–56.

Sunderland, A., Wade, D.T. and Hewer, R.L. (1987) The natural history of visual neglect after stroke, *International Disability Studies*, **9**, no. 2, 55–9.

Tepperman, P.S., Sovic, R. and Devlin, H.T.M. (1986) Stroke rehabilitation: A problem orientated approach, *Stroke*, **80**, no. 8, 158–67.

Thames, G. and McNeil, J.S. (1987) Independence levels and social adjustment of post-stroke patients, *Health and Social Work*, **Spring**, 121–5.

Thompson, S.B.N. (1982) Does Information Influence Affect the Interpretation of Photographic Stimuli with Human Content? *BA(Hons) Dissertation*, Psychology Dept., Plymouth Polytechnic, Plymouth, UK.

Thompson, S.B.N. (1983a) Training surface personnel: Implications from a recent study, *Nautical Magazine*, **229**, no. 4, 16–7.

Thompson, S.B.N. (1983b) Training influences on maritime personnel, *Nautical Magazine*, **230**, no. 3, 18–9.

Thompson, S.B.N. (1983c) Organised diversion can work against patients, *Therapy Weekly*, **10**, no. 1, 7.

Thompson, S.B.N. (1984a) Computer-assisted visual feedback as a potential prognostic tool for adult hemiplegia in Occupational Therapy, *Postgraduate Diploma in Information Systems Dissertation PD/20*, School of Information Science, Portsmouth Polytechnic, Portsmouth, UK.

Thompson, S.B.N. (1984b) Investigacion psicologica con personal de superficie de la marina, *La Revista Psicologia General y Aplicada*, 193–4.

Thompson, S.B.N. (1985a) The use of microcomputers to assist the recovery of stroke patients, *Paper presented at Postgraduate Diploma in Information Systems Seminars*, Portsmouth Polytechnic, Portsmouth, UK, 27th February 1985.

Thompson, S.B.N. (1985b) Computerised therapy for leg injuries, *Therapy Weekly*, **10**, no. 11, 4.

Thompson, S.B.N. (1986) Monitoring nerve impulses in leg muscles, *Therapy Weekly*, **13**, no. 15, 4.

Thompson, S.B.N. (1987a) A stochastic model of cerebrovascular accident prognosis. *PhD Thesis*, School of Information Science, Portsmouth Polytechnic, Portsmouth, UK.

Thompson, S.B.N. (1987b) A microcomputer-based assessment battery, data file handling and data retrieval system for the forward planning of treatment for adult stroke patients, *Journal of Microcomputer Applications*, **10**, no. 2, 127–35.

Thompson, S.B.N. (1987c) Using information systems technology in the assessment and prognosis of stroke patients in Occupational Therapy. *Paper presented at Postgraduate Diploma in Information Systems Seminars*, Portsmouth Polytechnic, Portsmouth, UK, 10th June, 1987.

Thompson, S.B.N. (1987d) A microcomputer-feedback system for improving control of incompletely innervated leg muscle in adult cerebrovascular accident patients, *British Journal of Occupational Therapy*, **50**, no. 5, 161–6.

Thompson, S.B.N. (1987e) Testing manual dexterity, *Therapy Weekly*, **3**, no. 38, 4.

Thompson, S.B.N. (1987f) A system for rapidly converting quadriceps contraction to a digital signal for use in microcomputer-oriented muscle therapy and stroke patient assessment schedules, *Computers in Biology and Medicine International Journal*, **17**, no. 2, 117–25.

Thompson, S.B.N. and Coleman, M.J. (1987a) A quantitative assessment of neuromuscular function for use with unilateral cerebrovascular accident patients, *International Journal of Rehabilitation Research*, **10**, no. 3, 312–6.

Thompson, S.B.N. and Coleman, M.J. (1987b) Making the therapists' prognosis of stroke a more scientific process, *Paper presented at First International Convention of Human Service Information Technology Applications (HUSITA 87)*, on A Technology to Support Humanity at City of Birmingham Polytechnic, Birmingham, UK, 7–11th September, 1987, in *Information Technology and Human Services* (1988) (eds B. Glastonbury, W. LaMendola and S. Toole), John Wiley, Chichester, pp. 68–75.

Thompson, S.B.N. and Coleman, M.J. (1987c) An interactive micro-computer-based system for the assessment and prognosis of stroke patients, *Paper presented at Special European Conference of the American Society for Cybernetics*, on Design for Development of Social Systems at University of St. Gallen, St. Gallen, Switzerland, 15–19th March, 1987, in *Journal of Microcomputer Applications*, (1989) **12**, no. 1, 33–40.

Thompson, S.B.N. and Coleman, M.J. (1987d) Leg-injured patients switch on to rehabilitation, *Therapy Weekly*, **13**, no. 48, 7.

Thompson, S.B.N. and Coleman, M.J. (1987e) An investigation into stroke, *Therapy Weekly*, **13**, no. 29, 7.

Thompson, S.B.N. and Coleman, M.J. (1987f) Occupational therapists' prognoses of their patients: Findings of a British survey of stroke, *International Journal of Rehabilitation Research*, (1988) **11**, no. 3, 275–9.

Thompson, S.B.N. and Coleman, M.J. (1987g) Stroke recovery model, *Therapy Weekly*, **14**, no. 9, 7.

Thompson, S.B.N., Coleman, M.J. and Yates, J. (1986) Visual feedback as a prognostic tool, *Journal of Microcomputer Applications*, **9**, no. 3, 215–21.

Thompson, S.B.N., Hards, B. and Bate, R. (1986) Computer assisted visual feedback for new hand and arm therapy apparatus, *British Journal of Occupational Therapy*, **49**, no. 1, 19–21.

Tieton, C.N. and Maloaf, M. (1982) Diagnosing the problems in stroke, *American Journal of Nursing*, **82**, 596–600.

Totara, G.J. and Anagnostakos, N.P. (1987) *Principles of Anatomy and Physiology*, 5th edn, Harper and Row.

Towle, J.A., Edmans, J.A. and Lincoln, N.B. (1988) Use of computer-presented games with memory-impaired stroke patients, *Clinical Rehabilitation*, **2**, 303–7.

REFERENCES

Triptree, V.J. and Harrison, M.A. (1980) The use of sensor pads in the treatment of adult hemiplegia, *Physiotherapy*, **66**, no. 9, 299.

Trombley, C.A. (1983) *Occupational Therapy for Physical Dysfunction*, 2nd edn, Williams and Wilkins, Baltimore.

Tuhrim, S. and Reggia, J.A. (1986) Feasibility of physician-developed expert systems, *Medical Decision Making*, **6**, no. 1, 23–6.

Turczynski, B.E., Hartje, W. and Sturm, W. (1984) Electromyographic feedback of chronic hemiparesis: An attempt to quantify treatment effects, *Archives in Physical Medicine Rehabilitation*, **65**, no. 9, 526–8.

Turner, A. (1987) *The Practice of Occupational Therapy*, Churchill Livingstone, London.

Turton, A.J. and Frazer, C.M. (1988) A test battery to measure the recovery of voluntary movement control following stroke, *British Journal of Occupational Therapy*, **51**, no. 1, 11–4.

Ullman, M. (1964) Disorders of body image after stroke, *American Journal of Nursing*, **64**, no. 10, 89–91.

Visser, S.L. and Aanen, A. (1981) Evaluation of EMG parameters for analysis and quantification of hemiparesis, *Electromyography and Clinical Neurophysiology*, **21**, 591.

Vodovnik, L. and Rebersek, S. (1973) Myoelectrical and myomechanical prehension systems using functional electric stimulation in control of upper extremity, in *Protheses and Orthoses*, (eds P. Herberts, R. Kadefors, R. Magnessum and I. Peterson), Charles Thomas, Springfield, Illinois, pp. 151–65.

Voss, D.E. (1959) Proprioceptive neuromuscular facilitation, *American Journal of Occupational Therapy*, **13**, no. 4, part 2, 191–4.

Voss, D.E. (1967) Proprioceptive neuromuscular facilitation, *American Journal of Physical Medicine*, **46**, no. 1, 838–98.

Voss, D.E. (1972) Proprioceptive neuromuscular facilitation: The PNF method, in *Physical Therapy Services in the Developmental Disabilities*, (eds) Pearson and Williams, Charles Thomas, Springfield, Illinois.

Wade, D.T. and Collin, C. (1988) The Barthel ADL Index: A standard measure of disability?, *International Disability Studies*, **10**, no. 2, 64–7.

Wade, D.T., Hewer, R.L., Skilbeck, C.E. and David, R.M. (1985) *Stroke – A Critical Approach to Diagnosis, Treatment and Management.*

Wade, D.T., Hewer, R.L., Wood, V.A. (1984a) Stroke: The influence of age on outcome, *Age and Ageing*, **13**, 357–62.

Wade, D.T., Hewer, R.L., Wood, V.A., Skilbeck, C. and Ismail, H.M. (1978) The hemiplegic arm after stroke: Measurement and recovery, *Journal of Neurological Neurosurgical Psychiatry*, **46**, 521.

Wade, D.T., Parker, V. and Hewer, R.L. (1986) Memory disturbances after stroke: Frequency and associated losses, *International Rehabilitation Medicine*, **8**, 65–8.

Wade, D.T., Skilbeck, C., Wood, V.A. and Hewer, R.L. (1984b) Long term survival after stroke, *Age and Ageing*, **13**, 76–82.

Walker, A.E., Robbins, M. and Weinfield, F.D. (1981) Clinical findings in *The National Survey of Stroke* (ed. F.D. Weinfield), *Stroke*, **12**, suppl. 1, 13–44.

Wall, J.C. and Ashburn, A. (1979) Assessment of gait disability in hemiplegics, *Scandinavian Journal of Rehabilitation Medicine*, **11**, 95–103.

Wall, P.D. (1980) Mechanisms of plasticity connection following damage in adult mammalian nervous systems, in *Recovery of Function: Theoretical Considerations for Brain Injury Rehabilitation* (ed. Bach-y-Rita), University Park Press, Baltimore, pp. 91–105.

Wallhagen, I. (1979) The split brain: Implications for care and rehabilitation, *American Journal of Nursing*, **79**, 2118–25.

Wannstedt, G.T. and Herman, R.M. (1978) Use of augmented sensory feedback to achieve symmetrical standing, *Physical Therapy*, **58**, 553–9.

Weiner, W.J. and Goetz, C.G. (1981) *Neurology for the Non-Neurologist*, Harper and Row, Philadelphia.

Weisberg, L.A. (1979) Computerised tomography and pure motor hemiparesis, *Neurology (NY)*, **29**, 490–5.

Whisnant, J.P. (1974) The decline of stroke, *Stroke*, **15**, 160–8.

Wiederhold, V. (1976) ARAMIS manual, *Project Report*, Dept. of Immunology, Stanford University Medical Center, Stanford.

Winchester, P., Montgomery, J., Bowman, B. and Hislop, H. (1983) Effects of feedback stimulation training and cyclical electrical stimulation on knee extension in hemiparetic patients, *Physical Therapy*, **63**, no. 7, 1096–103.

Winkler, R.L. (1972) *An Introduction to Bayesian Inference and Decision*, Holt, Rinehart and Winston, New York.

Wolf, S.L., Baker, M.P. and Kelly, J.L. (1979) EMG biofeedback in stroke: Effect of patient characteristics, *Archives in Physical Medicine Rehabilitation*, **60**, 96–102.

Wolf, S.L. and Binder-MacLeod, S.A. (1983) Electromyographic biofeedback applications to the hemiplegic patient. Changes in upper extremity neuromuscular and functional status, *Physical Therapy*, **63**, no. 9, 1393–1403.

Wolf, S.L. and Hudson, J.E. (1980) Feedback signal based upon force and time delay: Modification of the Krusen Limb Load Monitor, *Physical Therapy*, **60**, 1289–90.

Young, J.F. and Reid, M. (1972) Care in the surgical management of intracranial aneurysms, *Journal of Neurosurgical Nursing*, **4**, no. 7, 21–31.

Zagoria, R.J. and Reggia, J.A. (1983) Transferability of medical decision support systems based on Bayesian Classification, *Medical Decision Making*, **3**, no. 4, 501–9.

Index